These Aren't Just 20 essential supplements for super health
They're Essential for *Your* Health.

Did You Know That . . .

• There are sugars called *glyconutrients* that can stimulate your immune system, fight cancer and reduce heart disease? — *see page 93*

• Natural micronized progesterone has all the benefits of synthetic HRT drugs without the dangerous side effects? — *see page 183*

• Soy isoflavones can reduce your risk of heart disease, menopausal discomfort and osteoporosis? — *see page 139*

• Essential fatty acids, also called omega-3 fats, can protect your heart, fight arthritis and improve brain function? — *see page 43*

• Vitamin C battles the common cold and flu and plays a vital role in dozens of body processes and functions? — *see page 35*

• The herb astragalus, which has been used for centuries in Asian cultures, can dramatically increase your immune function and ability to fight infection? — *see page 87*

20 ESSENTIAL SUPPLEMENTS *for* SUPER HEALTH

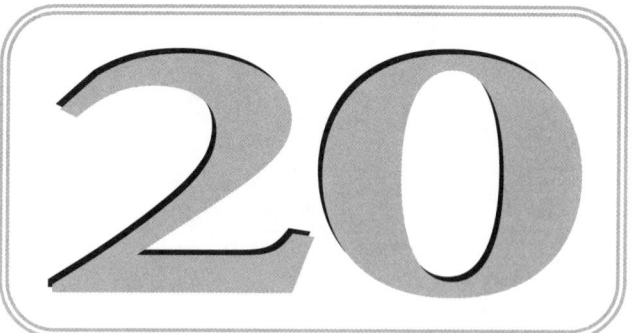

Essential Supplements *for* Super Health

Today's Can't-Do-Without Nutritional Supplements That Can Prevent Disease and Ultimately Save Your Life!

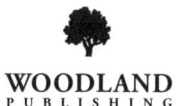

WOODLAND
PUBLISHING

Copyright © 2003 by Woodland Publishing
All rights reserved. No part of this publication may be reproduced, stored in a retrieval system, or transmitted in any form without the prior written permission of the copyright owner.

The CIP record for this book is available from the Library of Congress.

For ordering information, contact:
Woodland Publishing, P.O. Box 160, Pleasant Grove, Utah 84062
(800) 777-2665

Note: The information in this book is for educational purposes only and is not recommended as a means of diagnosing or treating an illness. All matters concerning physical and mental health should be supervised by a health practitioner knowledgeable in treating that particular condition. Neither the publisher nor author directly or indirectly dispenses medical advice, nor do they prescribe any remedies or assume any responsibility for those who choose to treat themselves.

ISBN 1-58054-359-6

Printed in the United States of America

Please visit our website:
www.woodlandpublishing.com

Contents

Essential Supplements: An Introduction 9

Chapter 1 Multivitamin-Mineral 19

Chapter 2 Vitamin C 35

Chapter 3 Essential Fatty Acids 43

Chapter 4 Vitamin B Complex 51

Chapter 5 Echinacea 69

Chapter 6 Probiotics: Beneficial Bacteria 77

Chapter 7 Astragalus 87

Chapter 8 Glyconutrients: Healthy Sugars 93

Chapter 9 Beta Carotene and Vitamin A 107

Chapter 10 Fiber 117

Chapter 11 Green Tea 125

Chapter 12 Coenzyme Q10 133

Chapter 13 Soy Isoflavones 139

Chapter 14 Garlic 147

Chapter 15 Olive Leaf Extract 153

Chapter 16 Saw Palmetto 161

Chapter 17 Calcium 167

Chapter 18 Grapeseed Extract 175

Chapter 19 Micronized Natural Progesterone 183

Chapter 20 "Green" and "Phyto" Foods 197

Chapter 21 Other Essential Supplements 207

Selected References 213
Index 217

Essential Supplements: An Introduction

UNTIL JUST A few years ago, most people considered vitamins and minerals somewhat strange and exotic, and herbs something that made pizza sauce a little more tasty. Nutritional supplements were found only in a few scattered health food stores, and those people interested in taking them were often regarded as health "nuts."

How things have changed. Today, more than 100 million Americans take some sort of nutritional supplement, whether it be a multivitamin/mineral, a homeopathic remedy for the flu, or an herbal preparation for migraine headaches. This means that close to half of our country's population is now regularly taking supplements to treat disease or to promote overall health.

Until recently, however, our choice of supplements was quite limited. For instance, most of the over-the-counter products available and widely used in Europe were simply not found in the United States due to restrictive laws. In response to growing consumer demand, Congress passed in 1994 the Dietary Supplement Health and Education Act (DSHEA), which has drastically changed the way nutritional supplements are produced, marketed and sold in this country. The law removed decades of regulatory barriers that had made it extremely difficult, if not impossible, to bring new products to market. For one thing, most supplements are derived from natural products, and natural products cannot be patented. Thus, pharmaceutical companies do not want to invest the hundreds of millions of dollars necessary for the testing and approval from the Food and Drug Administration (FDA) because they will never recoup their investment. The new set of laws declared nutritional supplements to be food products, and therefore not subject to the same expensive and (sometimes) rigorous testing normally required of new synthetic drugs by the FDA. As a result, many supplements that previously would have been classified as drugs and regulated by the FDA can now be sold over the counter in health food stores, pharmacies, and even your local grocery store.

Under the old set of laws, even products that had been used safely and effectively overseas for decades could not be used in the United States without undergoing the expensive testing required by the FDA for drugs. Under the current DSHEA codes, any product with a reasonable safety record can be quickly brought to market. So, if a product has been used for thousands of years by herbal healers in other cultures, or for decades in other countries where the product is regarded as safe, then that product can be produced and sold in this country without undergoing FDA approval. In fact, the FDA now has the responsibility to prove that a supplement is unsafe before it can pull the product off the shelves.

Another major change is that manufacturers are allowed some flexibility in making claims for health benefits of their particular supplement, as long as that claim is based on scientific evidence. For instance, if an herbal supplement has backing showing it can shorten the duration of colds, the manufacturers are allowed to say so on their labels and packaging.

Blessing or Burden?

On one hand, this new freedom in the supplement industry has been a boon to consumers. In 1995 alone, the first year after the new laws took effect, an astounding twenty thousand new supplements were introduced to the American marketplace. Each year since, thousands more have been introduced. A simple stroll through the aisles of any health food store clearly demonstrates the widespread effect the new regulations have had on the availability of nutritional supplements.

On the other hand, this new freedom in the marketplace has created an interesting dilemma for consumers, especially for those relatively new to natural health therapies such has herbal products or homeopathic remedies. One might argue that the more products are available, the more choice the consumer has, creating the ideal market, right? Not quite. The last eight years have produced a virtual avalanche of nutritional supplements, some that are manufactured with high-quality standards, some that aren't. Because there is no real governing body overseeing consistent standards in manufacturing, packaging, and shipping, there is no guarantee that you, the consumer, are actually getting what you paid for. And like any industry that presents opportunities of financial bounty, unscrupulous manufacturers, advertisers and marketers have misled consumers with a wide variety of miraculous health claims and unsubstantiated hype. Whether it's the daily paper, late-night infomercials, or website pop-up ads, there seems to be no shortage of amazing claims that a particular product can "fight cancer," "relieve PMS," "provide an amazing energy boost," or "give you the figure you've always wanted."

This is not to say that there aren't nutritional products that can actually deliver on these promises. The problem is that with each new product (and remember, we're talking about thousands of new ones every year) accompanied by various claims of health and happiness, many of today's consumers are left feeling overwhelmed with the uncertainty of which supplements they should be taking. It seems that only those relatively few individuals with the time and resources to educate themselves properly regarding the validity of each supplement and to wade through the incessant flow of health claims, could have a reasonable grasp of which supplements might provide real and lasting results.

Which Supplements Should I Take?

It is the current state of the nutritional supplement industry—the influx of thousands of new products yearly, accompanied by a barrage of advice, conflicting "expert" advice and promises of miraculous results—that sparked the idea for this book. With the shelves of health food stores and pharmacies literally teeming with new products, most people can only wonder, "Which supplement should I take?" With this in mind, we decided to construct a list of a relatively few supplements that are widely popular—and not only popular, but that provide health benefits which are real, wide-ranging, and backed by solid evidence. In other words, a list of supplements that are *essential* for overall good health and disease prevention?

The supplements discussed in this book contain nutrients that are crucial for the proper functioning of the human body. They provide wide-reaching benefits and are involved in varied and vital body functions. Of course, you could certainly educate yourself about the benefits of other legitimate supplements not covered here, and we would encourage you to do so. But for those who are simply left bewildered and overwhelmed by the flood of new supplements, overhyped products and contradictory advice, this book is your best bet to implementing a sound and practical supplement plan.

Things to Consider When Purchasing and Using Supplements

- An ideal multivitamin/mineral supplement will contain vitamin A, beta-carotene, vitamins C, D, E, and K, B-complex vitamins (B6, B12, thiamin, niacin, folic acid, pantothenic acid, biotin, riboflavin), calcium, magnesium, zinc, iodine, selenium, copper, manganese, chromium, molybdenum, and possibly iron.

- Most standard multivitamin/mineral products contain the minimum DRIs (formerly the RDAs) for the vitamins, while minerals are included at less than minimum amounts. For this reason, if you think you're not making up the balance of minerals in your diet, you may need to take a separate multimineral supplement, or separate mineral products.

- Remember that while following the DRIs provides a starting point, your individual needs will vary. For instance, pregnant women need at least twice as much iron, vitamin D and folic acid than other women. If you're nursing an infant, you need more of everything, especially calcium. In fact, you probably need more nutrients to stay healthy than you did while you were pregnant. Older people also need to change their thinking when it comes to supplements. Many seniors are deficient in calcium, the B vitamins, selenium and vitamin D. Simply stated, your age, sex, dietary habits and lifestyle all have a significant effect on your nutrient needs.

- When deciding when to take your supplements, generally speaking, taking them with food is a good rule of thumb to follow. This may help replicate the synergistic action of all the nutrients that may be present naturally in food when it is being digested and assimilated. Moreover, many people experience nausea when taking supplements on an empty stomach. Of course, make sure you read the label instructions and follow them accordingly.

- Make sure you keep all your supplements in a cool, dry place. Leaving them in a hot place, such as a car, or with their container unsealed, increases the risk of the supplement losing its potency. Keep supplements away from humid places (which include bathroom medicine cabinets), and avoid storing them over the stove or in places that are regularly exposed to sunlight.

- Look at the expiration date on your supplement bottle label. They may not be effective if used after this date. As a general rule, minerals are quite stable and do not degrade, even when stored for long periods of time. Vitamins are less stable, but can be stored for fairly long periods of time. Herbs vary widely, depending especially on their form (powder, tablet, capsule, liquid, and so forth). Make sure you check the expiration date on any supplement before you buy it.

- When it comes to herbal supplements, it's vital to ensure that your products have a guaranteed potency and offer standardized active ingredients. Sometimes, this may require a bit of homework on your part in the form of research on companies and their products. Asking a consultant in a health food store is a good place to start. There are many publications that list reputable manufacturers and their line of products.

- Make sure you are getting the ingredients you are looking for. This can be especially tricky with herbs, as there are numerous genera and species that may share a common name. If an herbal product does not list the genus and species on its label, do not buy the product.

- Follow the label instructions. Do not assume that more is always better.

- If you are prone to allergic reactions, are pregnant or nursing, or are taking other drugs for any condition, it is wise to consult with a qualified health care provider regarding any supplements you may wish to take.

- If you are considering taking any supplement as a form of therapy for a specific condition, you should consult with your health care provider. He or she will be able to provide direction and ensure safety while supervising your supplement regimen.

How to Use This Book

Most important to remember is that all of the nutritional supplements covered here have been studied extensively and are widely regarded as safe and effective, as long as they are used judiciously. For these reasons, any or all of them are excellent choices when considering ways that you can prevent disease and better your overall health.

Of course, none of these supplements alone can cure a particular disease nor dramatically improve one's health. That's why they are called supplements, not "replacements." Their purpose is not to replace a healthful, varied diet, only to supplement it.

When considering taking any of the supplements listed in the book, there are a few things to look for. Each chapter will have a "Fast Facts" sidebar that may list a number of things, including any special instructions, considerations regarding safety or side effects, and even the best food sources for each particular nutrient. Other sidebars in the chapters give pertinent, if not crucial, information regarding that nutrient. The remaining material in each chapter should provide you with the information necessary to decide if that particular supplement is right for you—types of products available, their specific benefits, which diseases they can help prevent, their history, and so forth.

So, if you're one of the many people frustrated and overwhelmed by the literal flood of new products, loud hype and contradictory advice surrounding nutritional supplements, this book is for you. Good luck, and good health!

1

Multivitamin-Mineral

OKAY. THIS IS IT. If you were to take only one of the many supplements available today, it should be a high-quality multivitamin-mineral supplement. Why? A good "multi" will provide you with a wide variety of nutrients—including many discussed in this book—that are necessary for the basic functioning of the human body, disease prevention and overall good health. Obviously there's no guarantee that you'll never get sick if you take a multivitamin. But if you're looking for good general help, then the multi is your best choice.

How important can a vitamin-mineral supplement be for you? Consider this: In 2002, the American Medical Association, normally a very conservative entity, published a recommendation for all adults to take a multivitamin-mineral supplement. Stating that it is probable that most of us are not receiving adequate levels of essential nutrients, the AMA recommended that all adults, and especially women and high-risk groups (such as the elderly and those with chronic conditions), take a multivitamin-mineral supplement.

Many of you may be thinking that there is nothing revolutionary about a multivitamin-mineral supplement. They've been around for a long time, we've all seen commercials for them on TV, and they've lined the shelves of grocery stores for years. Our recommendation to consider a high-quality multi comes in a time when there are literally thousands of products out there. The presence of so many enticing supplements, accompanied by a barrage of media coverage, magical health claims and slick infomercials, may have distracted many consumers from the basic, yet vital, benefits that a multivitamin can provide.

One important fact to remember is that no supplement—not even the best available multivitamin-mineral—can replace a healthful, varied diet. However, most experts are beginning to agree that it is nearly impossible to get all the nutrients that our bodies require. Many factors, including the huge numbers of food products that are refined and high in sugar and unhealthy fats, the incessant advertising of manufacturers for foods that are simply unhealthy, busier lifestyles, and lower-than-normal nutrient levels in whole foods (such as vegetables and fruits) make it very difficult for most of us to get desired amounts of needed nutrients.

So, our suggestion follows that of most experts—a high-quality multivitamin-mineral supplement may be the best health insurance your dollars can buy.

When considering many consumers who are taking supplements (especially consumers new to the supplement "experience") the best initial recommendation is to regularly take a complete multi. This makes sense for several reasons:

- It will just about guarantee that diets less than perfect will not put the individual at risk for micronutrient deficiencies.

- It will provide high levels of certain nutrients that are known to be beneficial at levels above what is possible to obtain from diet alone and what is higher than what the government recommends.

- Since it is often difficult to motivate many people to take supplements for longer than a few months, a single multivitamin-mineral represents a more simple behavior change than does a regimen of many different supplements or special diets.

- A good multi is especially necessary for individuals with increased needs, such as pregnant/lactating women, the elderly, those experiencing unusually high levels of stress, the chronically ill, individuals with compromised immune systems, and even vegetarians.

Choosing a Multivitamin-Mineral Supplement

When it actually comes time to choose a multivitamin-mineral supplement, the prospects can be daunting. You'll probably find literally dozens of different brands, several different forms (tablets, capsules, powders, liquids, etc.), varying ingredients, and a huge range in price. Don't despair. The following will give you a good idea of how to pick the multivitamin-mineral (and many other supplements, for that matter) that both suits your needs and fits your budget.

MULTIVITAMIN-MINERAL FAST FACTS

Product Forms: Tablets, capsules, liquid

Possible Benefits: Disease prevention of chronic and common conditions like heart disease, diabetes, arthritis; maintenance of basic body functions and processes; prevention of nutrient deficiencies

Special Instructions/Cautions: If you are seeking a multivitamin-mineral product for treatment of a specific disease, you should consult with your qualified health care provider to determine which product may best fit your needs.

Multivitamin-Mineral 23

- Decide where you want to purchase supplements from: You can find multivitamin-mineral supplements just about anywhere these days. Grocery stores, drugstore and pharmacy chains, internet sites and health food stores are prime examples. Regardless of where you choose to purchase your supplement, make sure the return policies of the retailer are to your satisfaction. You want to choose a retailer that has good turnover for the product. What that means is that you don't want to buy something that has been sitting on the shelf for two years. Check the expiration date. If it is expiring soon, you have to question if the product is not selling well (perhaps meaning consumers don't buy it because it doesn't work).

  Also, make sure you have a customer service friendly retailer. This means that if you have cracked tablets, a "clumpy" powder, or allergic reaction to the product, you are able return it for your money back.

- Consider various factors when looking at your budget. Do a little research, comparing the price range of the product you are considering. If you notice that most supplements are over ten dollars, and you find one that is only three dollars, then that is a good indication that product is probably inferior. Drugstores and pharmacies tend to carry mass-market brands as well as their own store brands. There prices tend to be less expensive than brands carried at health food stores. There are several reasons for the price differences (marketing, profit margins, cost of raw materials and production run sizes).

Remember that within the different brands there are always going to be price variations. Some companies have higher operating cost, faster machinery, or purchase higher quality of raw materials. Additionally, finished product costs are affected by the quality control and lab testing that a company does. Lab tests can costs several thousands of dollars per product, which could certainly add a few extra dollars to the product you're considering.

Also keep in mind that more expensive doesn't always mean better and cheaper doesn't always mean less effective. But if you compare several other products and do a little homework on the products you're looking at, you'll have a better chance of selecting a quality product.

- Search for brands that conduct quality control tests. It's comforting to know that the company verifies and tests their raw materials for identification (that way you know you're getting echinacea and not grass clippings). Look for products that test the product's purity (that it is not contaminated with heavy metals such as mercury or lead). You also want a brand that conducts a "Finish Product Test" and "Stability Test." If it says there is 500 mg vitamin C in the capsule, this means the company has actually tested that product batch and not relied on other calculations. There are also companies that test their products after a year or two to ensure they are still potent. Most companies/manufacturers have websites or a contact phone number on their product labels. It can

EAT YOUR FRUITS AND VEGETABLES...
AND TAKE YOUR VITAMINS

In June 2002, the American Medical Association announced their recommendation that all adults, in particular women, the elderly and those who are chronically ill, regularly take vitamin and mineral supplements. Their report indicated that intake of vitamins and minerals below optimal levels are a risk factor for chronic disease. It also indicated what many health and nutrition experts have been preaching for some time—that nutrient deficiencies are common in the general population, especially the elderly. Citing numerous links to diseases such as cancer, cardiovascular disease, and osteoporosis, the report states that "it appears prudent for all adults to take vitamin supplements." So don't just take our word for it—do yourself a favor and find a quality multivitamin-mineral product that fits your specific needs.

be very helpful to contact the company and inquire about the quality control tests they perform.

- Look for products that bear the USP logo. This logo, which means "United States Pharmacopia," tells you that the vitamin-mineral supplement has been tested and approved for its adequate dissolving. While there are excellent products that haven't been tested by the USP, it is one indicator that your product will dissolve properly, allowing for better absorption.

- Look at the labels and packaging. Choose a brand that has legible labels, a front panel with the name and quantity of the product, side panels with the ingredients and nutritional labeling information, contact phone number and/or address of the manufacturer, a lot number, expiration date and clear instructions. Also, it is wise to choose a product that lists out the quantity of the ingredients and not just an ingredient list.

- Choose a brand that the store staff recommends (in an educated manner). Believe it or not, this is a good sign that the product is high quality. The recommendation could be due to the feedback from other customers, or it's an indication of a company committed to educating its retailers and customers about its product. If you're not sure about which product to choose, don't be afraid to ask the store staff. It may also be helpful to consider a brand that has informational leaflets available to consumers or that has conducted clinical studies on their products.

What Should My Multi Have in It?

There are no perfect answers here. And your situation—whether you're a man, woman or child, your age, your dietary habits, and the like—will determine which product may work best for you. Also remember that it may be wise to take some of these nutrients as separate supplements since the multi will not always provide them in adequate amounts (for instance, calcium is usually only present in minimal amounts because it is a "bulky" agent and simply takes up too much room). The following will hopefully give you a pretty good idea of what to consider for general purposes.

Vitamin A/Beta-carotene: It's probably best to look for a product that has more beta-carotene than vitamin A. It's far less toxic and can be utilized by the body as needed. Moreover, it appears that beta-carotene has more anticancer power than the converted vitamin A.

Vitamin C: Vitamin C is another important antioxidant and should be supplied at levels well above the minimum requirements (60 mg). There is much debate about how much is the optimal amount. Some prominent researchers advocate taking huge amounts—tens of thousands of milligrams daily—while others suggest more moderate levels (700–1,500 a day). Higher daily intake may only temporarily raise blood levels of the vitamin, though this could be beneficial. If you are looking to take more than what your multivitamin provides, you can easily take vitamin C as a separate supplement.

Bioflavonoids: These are often found in multi formulas. They are thought to enhance the action of vitamin C, and

> **DO YOU NEED A TRACE MINERAL SUPPLEMENT?**
>
> Depending on your specific needs, the multivitamin-mineral supplement you end up purchasing may or may not include what are called *trace minerals*—such as molybdenum, vanadium or boron. While these are required by the body in very small amounts, there is mounting research that more and more of us are suffering from deficiencies from such nutrients. One option is to consider taking a trace mineral supplement. While you may not need to take one every day, taking it at least occasionally can ensure that you are covering your bases when it comes to trace minerals.
>
> Where do you find a trace mineral supplement? Probably not at the grocery store, but you can generally find a good trace mineral product at your local health food store. And the good news is that they're fairly inexpensive.

research shows they are able to reduce the risk of certain diseases. Desired amounts are debatable, however.

Vitamin E: Vitamin E is an important antioxidant and should be supplied at levels well above the RDI of 30 IU/day. Many authorities recommend 200–1,000 IU per day for the prevention of age-related degenerative diseases such as cancer and atherosclerosis. Most natural health care providers prefer the natural d-alpha form of the vitamin, though there is still debate among which form is best.

Vitamin K: This has only recently been added to some multi formulas due to emerging evidence that it can prevent bone loss. Until more research is available, a daily dose of 80–300 mcg conforms to current RDI standards and normal dietary intakes. Supplementation with this vitamin is especially important to patients with a history of chronic antibiotic therapy or intestinal malabsorption.

Vitamin B Complex: This is a somewhat misunderstood group of vitamins. Each member is a separately functioning coenzyme in wide-ranging processes and functions of human biochemistry. If a customer has a specific condition for which a single B vitamin is known to be helpful, then a separate supplement of this vitamin may be added to the multivitamin-mineral regimen, preferably after consultation with a knowledgeable health provider. See the chapter on the B-complex vitamins in this book for optimal dosage amounts.

Vitamin D: For those patients who do not get regular exposure to sunlight or vitamin D fortified foods, 400 IU per day may be an optimal supplemental intake. However, individuals with increased risk for osteoporosis may benefit from as much as 800 IU per day. Finally, vitamin D deficiency has been recently linked to higher risks of colorectal and breast cancer, so it may now be more important to guarantee an adequate intake of vitamin D.

Calcium: Calcium is a problematic element in multivitamin-mineral formulas because it is so bulky. To provide adequate amounts of calcium would require a multivitamin to have a daily dosage of roughly six tablets—a number that often discourages a consumer from buying that particular product. Thus, many manufacturers attempt to reduce daily tablet requirements by lowering the calcium content in the daily total. So that means that you will probably need to take calcium as a separate supplement to get the optimal levels, especially if you are a woman. Also look for products that contain a calcium-citrate form.

Magnesium: Magnesium is essential for the use of calcium as the two share a common absorption pathway. And while too much magnesium can actually inhibit the absorption of calcium, and vice-versa, this only happens if one is present in largely disproportionate amounts. There is no real evidence that one form of magnesium is better absorbed than any other.

Potassium: Potassium is often included in multivitamin-mineral supplements at doses around 100 mg per tablet, far below a recommended intake of 3,000 mg or more. Clearly this amount is insignificant, but it appears to be illegal (by FDA ruling) for manufacturers to include more than this amount. However, individuals with varied, healthful diets usually don't have a problem receiving adequate amounts of potassium.

Zinc and Copper: These two work interdependently within the human body, so supplements should not contain large amounts of one at the expense of the other. A fifteen-to-one zinc-copper ratio is considered ideal with a range of 10 to 30 parts zinc to one part copper being acceptable.

Manganese: Manganese has received a lot of attention for its role in bone and joint health. Most supplements provide only a few milligrams, which satisfies the minimum requirements. You may want to look for a product that provides more than the minimum or consider taking a separate trace mineral supplement.

Chromium: Chromium is important in sugar and lipid metabolism and should be present in any complete multivitamin-mineral formula. However, some manufacturers include far less than the recommended 50–200 micrograms in their product's daily dose. Organically bound chromium (any available form except chloride) is known to be much better absorbed than inorganic chromium chloride. While there has been recent debate over the merits of chromium picolinate versus other forms of chromium for certain conditions, it has never been shown to be better for general nutrition purposes.

Selenium: This recently emerging nutrient has been identified as an important antioxidant cofactor and may be important in cancer prevention. A new RDI has been established at 70 mcg per day, but many formulas contain as much as 200 mcg per daily dose, which is in the upper range of recommended intakes according to some authorities. Inorganic selenium appears to be as available for absorption and metabolism as is organically combined selenium.

Other nutrients: Multivitamin-mineral products will vary widely in their make-up. Many include other trace minerals such as boron, molybdenum and vanadium. While there are no established recommendations for these nutrients, we do know they are necessary to some degree. If your multi product doesn't contain some of the trace minerals, you may want to consider taking an occasional trace mineral supplement (see the sidebar "Do You Need a Trace Mineral Supplement?"). This will ensure that you are receiving some of these essential nutrients, even in small amounts. Many products may also contain ingredients such as herbs, enzymes, probiotics, etc. There is wide disagreement as to whether they are helpful in these products. Our opinion is that they only add to the "bulk" of the product (thereby increasing the size and/or quantity of pills you have to take) and probably aren't present in amounts needed to provide significant benefits.

The Bottom Line

Like the opening of this chapter says, if you were to take only one supplement listed in this book, a good multivitamin-mineral would probably be your best bet. Chances are neither you nor I are getting optimal levels of all the nutrients we need just for basic body functions. That's why a multivitamin-mineral product can literally be a lifesaver—or at least a life prolonger. A good multi can make up for some of the lack we experience in our diet. The multivitamin-mineral supplement could now take the place of the apple in the old adage, "An apple a day keeps the doctor away."

2

Vitamin C

WHAT IF YOU could take one pill to promote healthy teeth, bones and other tissues, enhance immune function, promote healthy blood cell production, aid in adrenal gland function, fight free-radical production, prevent/treat urinary tract infections, help reduce cholesterol levels, and fight the common cold, among other things? Sound too good to be true? It's not—it's vitamin C. That's right, the vitamin you know is found in oranges, tomatoes and other citrus fruits—the one that you probably knew was generally good for you.

Well, decades of research have essentially etched in stone the myriad of health benefits offered by this marvelous vitamin. And undoubtedly more research will only reveal additional benefits.

VITAMIN C FAST FACTS

Possible Uses: heart disease, recovery from surgery, chronic inflammatory diseases (such as lupus and rheumatoid arthritis), bacterial/viral infections (including colds, influenza and urinary tract infections), fatigue, depression, degenerative disorders, cancer, gingivitis, asthma, allergies, angina, cataracts, sunburn, diabetes-related organ damage, high cholesterol, menopausal disorders, toxin exposure

Special Instructions: Take larger amounts in several doses of less than 1,000 mg each throughout the day. Make sure to take with adequate water. Smokers and those exposed to cigarette smoke, diabetics, sufferers of heart disease, cancer patients, and those with chronic inflammation and suppressed immune function can especially benefit from increased intake of vitamin C.

Dietary Sources: cabbage, citrus fruits, red/green bell peppers, strawberries, broccoli, Brussels sprouts, chili peppers, collard and turnip greens, guava, kale, parsley

Safety Issues: Safe at a wide range of doses. If you experience diarrhea when taking large amounts, cut back until the diarrhea subsides. Also, consuming large amounts of vitamin C can interfere with certain health tests, such as those testing for blood in the stool and sugar in the urine.

Getting Our C Rations

Before the late 1700s, sailors who joined the crew of a seagoing vessel knew that they had roughly a 50 percent chance of surviving their voyage. They weren't in danger of falling off the edge of the earth or being devoured by a sea monster. Instead, one of the greatest risks was that they might fall prey to a dreadful, and often deadly, disease that would make their gums bleed, their teeth fall out, cause bruising all over the body, and ultimately, kill them.

At that time, no one knew that this disease was scurvy, caused by a deficiency of vitamin C. On long trips, the ship's cook usually went through the fresh vegetables and fruit first, then served grains and meat, which contained little, if any, vitamin C until arriving at port. This meant that the crew would often go for long periods—often months—without this essential vitamin.

Eventually, it was discovered that oranges, lemons and limes could prevent this terrible disease, and British sailors were among the first to take along mandated rations of lime juice; hence their traditional nickname "limeys." It wasn't until the middle of this century that vitamin C was isolated as the component that protected against scurvy. Its scientific name, ascorbic acid, reflects its anti-scurvy past.

These days, most of us get enough vitamin C in our diets and never have to worry about scurvy. Many of us even keep extra bottles of vitamin C on hand so we can down a few hundred milligrams if we feel a cold coming on. Or we may occasionally take a multivitamin/mineral supplement that contains extra vitamin C. In fact, vitamin C is one of the top-selling supplements in this country, mainly because of its cold and flu-fighting capabilities. However, that's just one of its many vital roles in the human body.

Building the Body

One of vitamin C's most crucial tasks is to help in the formation of collagen, the fibrous protein that comprises the principal structural tissue in the body. In other words, it is one of the main components that holds us together.

In simple terms, vitamin C is involved in the processes that allow tissue fibers to "weave" together and become stronger. When these fibers don't link or weave together, we experience the symptoms typical of scurvy. Remember what early sailors experienced with the onset of scurvy? Bleeding gums, teeth falling out, bleeding under the skin. In essence, we begin to fall apart. And since collagen is a primary agent in healing damaged tissues, these things only get worse, not better.

And it's not just scurvy symptoms that we need to worry about. A low intake of vitamin C can also worsen the symptoms of osteoporosis, cancer and heart disease. But more on those later.

Free Radical Fighter

The mountains of research done on vitamin C, especially lately, shows that it is a potent fighter of free radicals, or oxidants, which initiate chemical reactions that lead to the breakdown of cells and tissues. There are normal processes of the body that involve oxygen—namely, that of oxygen being carried via the bloodstream to every cell in the body—where it is used for metabolizing energy. This process potentially can lead to the creation of molecular particles, generally known as free radicals. These molecules lack an electron, making them unstable and leading them to "steal" an electron from some other molecule. That molecule is then lacking an electron and becomes a free radical, continuing this free radical domino effect.

Vitamin C aids in halting this cycle of thievery. How? It can surrender one of its electrons without becoming a dangerous free radical, thus stopping a whole string of "electron-stealing." This is important because damage resulting from free radicals is widely thought to be involved in many diseases and degenerative conditions, including heart disease, aging, cancer, inflammation, viral infections and more.

As an antioxidant or free radical fighter, vitamin C improves the functioning of various areas of the body. For instance, vitamin C can help us breathe better because it protects against the many and varied toxins that we inhale every day. In addition, immune cells use a lot of oxygen when going about their tasks, which can produce extra potentially damaging oxidants. However, if enough vitamin C is available, body tissues and cells are protected. Vitamin C also helps protect liver cells as they aid in the breakdown of toxins. And the list goes on and on.

MEGADOSING: HELPFUL OR HARMFUL?

A growing number of physicians and other health experts recommend the so-called "megadosing" of vitamin C and other supplements. Megadosing involves the consumption of amounts far higher than recommended daily values to the point of literally "flooding" or saturating the body with the vitamin, especially during times of illness.

So what is the rationale behind this practice? As discussed earlier, many illnesses involve damage from free radicals, unstable molecules that adversely affect healthy cells and tissues. Once started, this damage transforms itself into a chain reaction that quickly depletes areas of vitamin C, thus allowing the damage to spread even more.

To prevent this, some recommend saturating the body's tissues with unusually high amounts of vitamin C, enough to satiate damaged tissues and stop the oxidant chain reaction. Admittedly, there are numerous practitioners who profess to successfully using megadosing of vitamin C, often in the form of ascorbic acid, to fight conditions from the common cold to viral hepatitis. (Well-known health author James Balch, M.D., reports that he takes 2,000 mg daily, whether or not he is sick.)

One common recommendation is to take enough of the vitamin to produce loose stools (often called "bowel tolerance"), then reduce the amount until the stools become more normal. The thinking is that these high doses of vitamin C will actually be utilized by the sick individual, thus they are able to tolerate the high doses. For instance, someone with a bad cold could take anywhere from one to ten grams of vitamin C two or three times an hour until they reach bowel tolerance. Depending on the person and the severity of their condition, the amount and time frame will vary, but tolerance could occur within four to eight hours. When that point is reached, many people find that their symptoms quickly vanish or are drastically diminished. And depending on the sickness, the megadosing could continue for a few days (for the flu or cold) or indefinitely (for chronic conditions like hepatitis).

Of course, the scientific backing for the practice of megadosing is mixed. And the research that has been done only focuses on a limited number of health conditions. Before starting a megadosing therapy, it would be wise to consult with your health care physician.

The Energy Vitamin

One overlooked aspect of vitamin C's health repertoire is that of helping the body efficiently produce energy. It is required for the synthesis of a compound called carnitine, which aids in the transport of fatty acids into the mitochondria—the power plants of cells. While it's true that carbohydrates provide the building blocks of energy for most parts of our body, fatty acids are the primary sources for energy production in the skeletal muscles and the heart. You can imagine that if you don't have enough vitamin C, and thus enough carnitine, your heart and skeletal muscles will suffer from fatigue.

The Bottom Line

No doubt about it—vitamin C is not just helpful, it is crucial for the proper functioning of our body. And while it may be going overboard to "megadose," the indications are that taking more than the RDA—even as little as 200 mg or more daily—can produce significant results. Whether it is used for heart disease, gingivitis or fighting the flu, vitamin C is one of our body's premier health agents. So, if you're looking for a bona-fide, tried-and-true supplement with wide-reaching applications, vitamin C is one of your best bets.

3

Essential Fatty Acids

LATELY, YOU MAY have heard of a kind of "good" fat that can lower risk for heart disease, improve brain function, fight arthritis and other inflammatory diseases, and enhance immune function. These "good" fats are omega-3 fatty acids, which over the last several years have been shown to offer a variety of impressive benefits.

Like some types of fish, whales and other marine mammals are high in omega-3 polyunsaturated fatty acids (sometimes called PUFAs). Doctors and researchers working in the Arctic were among the first to discover the heart-healthy benefits of omega-3 fatty acids when they were investigating why the Innuit Eskimos, who normally dined on a diet high in fat and cholesterol of whale, seal and fish, rarely developed heart disease.

Subsequent studies in Greenland and elsewhere have confirmed that the rate of heart disease among the Inuit people was much lower than that of westerners, despite the fact that their diet was typically higher in fat.

The same studies that were done with omega-3 fatty acids in fish oils apply to the health benefits of omega-3 fatty acids from plant sources, most notably that of

---

ESSENTIAL FATTY ACID FAST FACTS

Product Forms: Omega-3 fatty acids, EPA (eicosapentaenoic acid), DHA (docosahexaenoic acid), flaxseed oil, EFAs (essential fatty acids)

Possible Benefits: Heart disease, arthritis, angina, high blood pressure, atherosclerosis, high cholesterol, asthma, breast cancer, colon cancer, lupus, multiple sclerosis, gout, migraines, rheumatoid arthritis, inflammatory conditions, suppressed immunity, osteoarthritis, dermatitis, sciatica, constipation, irritable bowel syndrome, stroke

Dietary Sources: Mackerel, salmon, bluefish, herring, albacore, rainbow trout, flaxseed

Possible Side Effects: Because of blood-thinning capabilities of fish oils, increased bleeding time may result, as well as more frequent nosebleeds and easy bruising. Do not take if you have a bleeding disorder or are on anticoagulants or are allergic to any kind of fish. Diabetics need be careful with fish oils. Flaxseed is generally regarded as safe.

flaxseed. Flax is the richest source of alpha linolenic acid (ALA). Like the omega-3 fatty acids found in fish oils, this fatty acid is necessary for the body to produce different compounds that help regulate blood pressure, clotting and other important functions.

Not All Fats Are Created Equal

The human body can produce most of the fat it needs from carbon, hydrogen and oxygen atoms found in food. But it doesn't have any way to create omega-3 and omega-6 fatty acids, the other types of fatty acids. Both of these belong to a category of fats called essential fatty acids (EFAs), and they come from only certain foods.

There are two varieties of omega-3. The first group is made up of eicosapentaenoic acid (EPA) and docosahexaenoic acid (DHA), which are found primarily in marine fish and mammals. The second type of omega-3s is ALA, found plant sources such as flaxseed. Once inside your body, some ALA can be converted into DHA and EPA for use.

The other essential fats that the body can't manufacture are the omega-6s, or linoleic acid. While omega-6 fats are vital to our health, most of us are probably getting too much of it in our diet. Most vegetable oils today are very high in omega-6 fats and low in omega-3 fats, causing an imbalance that could cause problems for our health. Most scientists believe that in the diets of our ancestors, the ratio of the two types of fats was nearly one to one. Today, the omega-6/omega-3 ratio is nearly ten to one.

How Do Essential Fats Help the Body?

Our bodies use both omega-3s and omega-6s to create a variety of short-lived substances called eicosanoids. These substances are amazing and crucial tools that our bodies use to perform many different functions, including regulating blood pressure, inducing blood clotting, controlling vital aspects of the reproductive cycle, among other things.

Prostaglandins, one of the better-known eicosanoids, are involved in nearly every body function, including those of the digestive, nervous and reproductive systems. They also have an effect on the brain, blood vessel walls, certain types of blood cells and blood platelets.

One potential problem with eicosanoids is that if there are too many omega-6 acids in the system and not enough omega-3s, conditions such as excessive blood clotting and narrowing of the arteries can result. However, if EPA and DHA (which are omega-3 fats found primarily in fish sources) are increased, they can decrease the stickiness of blood platelets involved in clotting, thus reducing the risk of a clot that could lead to a heart attack.

Additionally, the ALA content of flax and other plants can help reduce the risk of stroke by reducing the stickiness of blood platelets, which can lead to hardening of the arteries, stroke and heart attack. ALA can also help lower levels of triglycerides LDL cholesterol (the harmful variety). Finally, ALA has been shown to possess an anti-inflammatory effect that can help fight a number of illnesses, such as arthritis, irritable bowel syndrome and asthma, among others.

The Health Benefits of EFAs

The Heart/Cardiovascular System

There are piles of research detailing how omega-3 fats can lower blood pressure, decrease levels of triglycerides and LDL cholesterol, increase HDL cholesterol, lessen the risk of heart attack, stroke and related vascular disorders. There is also evidence that fish consumption may make heart attacks less dangerous if they do happen.

How do they do this? As mentioned previously, omega-3s can reduce the risk or even severity of heart disease by influencing several factors, including blood clotting and blood pressure. There is also mounting evidence showing that omega-3s can protect the heart against arrhythmias (wild fluctuations in the heartbeat caused by electrical malfunction), which can ultimately lead to death. This is an exciting area of research due to the large number of people who die each year from cardiac arrhythmia.

Arthritis

There are various studies focusing on the anti-arthritis effects of fish oils and other omega-3s. Most of these focus

> ## TYPES OF SUPPLEMENTS
>
> Essential fatty acids are sold under a variety of names, especially the fish oil products. They may be called fish oil, omega-3 fats, EFA's, or under the specific oil names such as DHA or EPA. Chances are, most fish oil products will probably contain a mixture of DHA and EPA, no matter what they're called. When in doubt, simply look for the ingredient label to see what the product contains.
>
> Regarding flaxseed products, these will vary as well. There are liquid and gelatin capsules (however, you may want to skip these and just add flaxseed to your diet due to the anticancer properties of lignans that are taken out when the oil is processed). Flaxseed oil may be seen simply by itself, or may be mixed with other omega-3 fatty acids in a combination product. Again, if you are in doubt, check the label for ingredients.

on rheumatoid arthritis, the joint-attacking kind that can begin even as early as childhood. A review of the ten best-conducted trials revealed that taking fish-oil supplements for at least three months resulted in modest but significant improvement, mainly morning stiffness and tenderness in joint areas. Other studies indicate that eating two or more servings of fish a week had about half the risk of developing rheumatoid arthritis as women who ate only one serving per week.

Cancer and Other Benefits

Omega-3 fatty acids may prove beneficial in other areas. Research indicates that they may help in preventing and treating certain cancers. In one study, researchers had twenty-five women with breast cancer eat a low-fat, high-fiber diet and take 10,000 mg of fish-oil supplements daily (which is far more than anyone would take under normal circumstances. After three months, the omega-3s stored in the women's breasts increased. This is important because other studies show that omega-3s delay the development of cancer and can inhibit tumor growth. Other research provides evidence that consuming dosages of omega-3s around 2,500 mg a day can prevent the abnormal cell proliferation that is linked with the risk of polyps and colon cancer.

What are some other health conditions for which omega-3s can help. Researchers are looking into the links between fish oil and reducing childhood asthma, helping women have healthier pregnancies (and thus healthier infants), improving bone growth, and lengthening remission for patients with Crohn's disease (a chronic inflammatory gastrointestinal disorder) who are already in prolonged remission. Some experts also believe that essential fatty acids can help lower the chances of and/or the severity of depression and related nervous system disorders.

The Bottom Line

Essential fatty acids provide the body with vital building blocks that affect nearly every body system. From cancer prevention to battling arthritis to promoting heart health, these "good" fats can do wonders in disease prevention and treatment. Additionally, science supports the varied and wide-reaching benefits of fish oils and flaxseed oil, making them some of today's most valuable and popular dietary supplements.

4

Vitamin B Complex

WE'VE ALL HEARD of B vitamins, often packaged as "vitamin B complex." Yet most of us probably take these essential nutrients for granted, because if we had a complete comprehension of how crucial they are to our well-being, we would go to great lengths to make sure we consumed them in adequate amounts.

Think of the B vitamins as little wooden blocks that build a tower. If one of these pieces is missing, the entire tower can crumble or is in danger of crumbling. Only working together can these separate building blocks attain their ultimate goal of building the tower.

Each individual B vitamin is important—vital, even. But you have to see the whole to understand the parts, and you have to understand the parts to appreciate the whole. It may also be tough for many people to even figure out what the parts are since there are quite a few, and many go by letters and numbers (B12, B6, etc.) while some go by their names (thiamin, riboflavin, etc.). It can be daunting.

Eight Vitamins for a Thousand Functions

The vitamin B family is comprised of eight members. All the B vitamins are water soluble, which means that they will dissolve in water. This is important because solubility affects your body's ability to absorb vitamins. Like vitamin C and other water-soluble vitamins, the B vitamins are absorbed directly into your bloodstream. Fat-soluble vitamins are not.

Working in concert, the B vitamins are a fascinating lot in that they are all necessary for the metabolism of proteins, fats and carbohydrates. While you may need individual B vitamins for specific reasons, taking them together is beneficial because each of them helps the others perform their duties. Like the example of a tower built of wood blocks, if one of the B vitamins is missing, then other B vitamins cannot carry out their duties. For instance, a lack of riboflavin will inhibit the performance of vitamin B6, preventing it from changing into coenzyme form.

In short, the eight B vitamins perform thousands of functions. The role they most often take is that of a sort of "helper-outer." In less-than-technical terms, these vitamins take part in the creation of coenzymes that assist in metabolism. These coenzymes assist enzymes, the protein catalysts that help initiate most of the vital reactions that occur in the body. Some B vitamins facilitate energy-releasing reactions, while others aid in the building of new cells that transport and deliver nutrients to other cells.

These functions benefit the body in myriad ways. Among their many benefits, B vitamins help alleviate menstrual and PMS complaints, prevent depression, regulate heart function, lower blood levels of homocysteine, prevent dysfunction of the nervous system, and prevent (or lessen) the effects of diabetes, to name just a few. The rest of this chapter will detail the health benefits of each of the B vitamins.

Vitamin B6 (Pyridoxine)

As is the case with various vitamins, vitamin B6 is comprised of more than one substance—in this case, three chemically similar components: pyridoxine, pyridoxal and pyridoxamine. All three of these substances are (or should be) present in almost all body tissues, with a high concentration in the liver. Of the three forms, pyridoxine is the most resistant to food processing and storage conditions, and is probably the form you are receiving most through your diet.

If you were to make up a list of the health conditions that each vitamin and mineral is supposed to help prevent or alleviate, the list for vitamin B6 would most likely be the longest. It is involved in dozens of physiologic activities, many of them vital. Vitamin B6 plays a primary role in protein metabolism, helps form hemoglobin, aids the absorption of amino acids from the intestine, and participates in the metabolizing of fats and carbohydrates. Additionally, scientists and health experts have established deficiencies of vitamin B6 with a wide variety of health conditions, including the following:

- ***Central nervous system breakdown.*** Vitamin B6 helps with energy transformation in the brain and nerve tissue. If it is deficient, convulsive seizures and related problems can result.

- ***Carpal tunnel syndrome.*** A lack of vitamin B6 has been shown to be involved in the onset of carpal tunnel syndrome. Additionally, supplementing with the vitamin has provided promising results for reversing and relieving the effects of the painful syndrome.

- ***Diabetes.*** If you have diabetes, you should seriously consider taking vitamin B6 supplements. Why? Diabetics experience less of the numbness and tingling of diabetes-related nerve damage if they receive extra B vitamins, especially B6.

- ***Heart disease.*** Along with other B vitamins, vitamin B6 is needed to break down a potentially toxic amino acid byproduct called homocysteine, of which high levels have been indicted in the progression of various forms of heart disease.

- ***Hormone regulation.*** Research shows that B6 has a

definitive role in regulating the actions of such hormones as estrogen, progesterone, androgen and glucocorticoid (a stress hormone). Though not known for sure, this may be why the vitamin often helps women with severe PMS and morning sickness symptoms.

- *Autism.* Though more research is needed, a number of studies indicate that megadoses of vitamin B6 may improve the condition of autistic people.

- *Kidney stones.* Research has linked B6 deficiencies with the formation of kidney stones.

Vitamin B12 (Cobalamin)

Like vitamin B6, vitamin B12 isn't just one substance. It's actually several compounds, all of which contain cobalt, giving them the generic name of cobalamins. And its complexity doesn't end there—it has the distinct honor of having the largest and most complicated chemical structure of any of the known vitamins.

One interesting note about vitamin B12 is that it cannot be synthesized by plants, which is why it is found primarily in meat and meat products. This is why vegetarians often have problems with vitamin B12 deficiencies. Additionally, vitamin B12 is the only vitamin that requires specific compounds from your digestive juices to be absorbed, which turns its absorption time from what is normally only a few seconds for other water-soluble vitamins to about three hours. Moreover, vitamin B12 is quite potent and durable, and foods containing B12 lose only about 30 percent of the vitamin when it is cooked.

Vitamin B12 is necessary for the proper function of every cell in your body. It is needed for DNA and RNA synthesis, the processes by which your body creates the genetic material that comprises the cell nucleus. Extra vitamin B12 is needed in areas where cells have a rapid turnover, such as the blood and intestines. When the vitamin is in short supply, cells can no longer divide and multiply. In the blood, it can mean anemia (a shortage of red blood cells) since cells in the bone marrow that make the red blood cells normally crank them out at a rate of about two hundred million a minute. In the intestines, it can mean a reduction in the absorption of nutrients, potentially leading to other nutrient deficiencies. These problems can be exacerbated by a lack of red blood cells, which help deliver specific nutrients to cells throughout the body.

Of course, there are other areas of which vitamin B12 can be of help. These include the following:

- ***Central nervous system problems.*** Various problems have been linked to a lack of vitamin B12, including memory loss, confusion, delusion, fatigue, loss of balance, numbness and tingling in the hands, ringing in the ears, and decreased reflexes. It has also been linked with multiple sclerosis-like symptoms and dementia. Research shows that vitamin B12 helps maintain the fatty sheath (called myelin) that surrounds and protects nerve fibers and promotes their normal growth. If the myelin breaks down due to B12 deficiency, nerve damage results, which can then cause or contribute to the before-mentioned nervous system problems.

- ***Homocysteine imbalance.*** Research indicates that a B12 deficiency raises the levels of homocysteine, which has been suggested as a cause of heart disease, heart attack and stroke and is toxic to the brain (which has raised questions regarding its role in the progression of Alzheimer's and other related disorders).

- ***Cancer prevention.*** In some areas of the body, such as the cervix and intestines, a shortage of B12 can begin to interfere with cell growth; the resulting cell abnormalities can eventually lead to cancer.

- ***Immune dysfunction.*** Your ability to fight infection may be reduced with deficiencies of vitamin B12 because your body can't produce enough white blood cells. Research shows that high levels of B12 in HIV-infected people can delay the development of full-blown AIDS.

Folic Acid (Folate)

An easy way to remember the best sources for this B vitamin is to think "foliage." In its food form, folate, folic acid was discovered by researchers after they waded through about four tons of spinach in order to isolate it.

Obviously, you won't need to eat four tons of spinach to get an adequate intake of folic acid, but spinach and other green leafy vegetables are some of its best food sources. Like other B vitamins, folic acid is necessary for a variety of functions and body processes, from cellular maintenance to the prevention of birth defects in developing fetuses.

Folic Acid and Genetic Engineering

Folic acid, like its B vitamin cousins, is essential for the synthesis of DNA and RNA. This means that it has to be readily available for your body to create the genetic blueprint that permits cells to properly develop and divide into other cells. If folic acid is in short supply, then the body has problems creating DNA and redistributing RNA (a sort of copy of the DNA needed for development of specific cell parts). The overall process slows the cells' ability to divide and multiply normally, thereby creating the potential for major, body-wide problems. For instance, in the blood, a deficiency can cause anemia, and in the intestinal tract it creates problems with nutrient absorption. More and more research is linking folic acid deficiencies to heart disease. And as you may know, doctors recommend that pregnant women take folic acid in order to prevent various birth defects.

Cancer Prevention with Folic Acid

Many factors can contribute to cancer—one in particular, damaged DNA, plays a pivotal role. Smoking, exposure to harmful chemicals from our environment and diet, exposure to x-rays, and certain viruses can all contribute to damaged cell DNA. When combined with a shortage of folic acid, which is vital to the creation and maintenance of the cell's genetic material, these risk factors can put you on the fast-track to cancer.

As mentioned earlier, folic acid deficiencies have been strongly indicted in the damage of cell DNA. In fact, a University of California Berkeley study found that even a mild shortage caused a large increase in the amount of damaged DNA. Other studies have linked folic acid deficiencies to the development of dysplasia (abnormal cell development, often linked to cancer) in the colon, lungs and cervix.

How Much Folic Acid Do We Need?

More research is coming to light that demonstrates how crucial folic acid is for our health, yet most of us aren't getting enough in our diets. On average we consume about 200 mcg daily (only half of the daily recommendation, which many experts believe is still inadequate). If this is true, it could bring about disastrous consequences, especially for women who are planning on getting pregnant or already are. Good food sources of folic acid are green leafy vegetables, lentils, pinto, navy, lima and kidney beans, tuna, oranges, strawberries, wheat germ, asparagus, bananas and cantaloupe. And it's important to eat these foods as fresh as possible, because heat and long storage times can destroy large amounts of folic acid content.

Pantothenic Acid

Like other B vitamins, pantothenic acid is involved in various body functions and processes—in fact, they number more than a hundred. It helps with the energy creation process and the production of fats, steroids, hormones, neurotransmitters and hemoglobin. Moreover, pantothenic acid is very common—so much so that its name comes from the Greek root *pantos*, which means "everywhere."

Pantothenic Acid and Coenzyme A

To understand how pantothenic acid could be involved in so many different bodily functions, it's important to know that it serves as an essential component of a substance called coenzyme A. Enzymes jump-start many chemical reactions that keep our bodies operating (in tip-top shape, hopefully).

Coenzyme A plays an extremely broad role, especially in the production of energy. It aids in the transportation of glucose, fatty acids and proteins as they are needed in the production of energy sources. We also use coenzyme A to detoxify the many chemicals that we may regularly take in our bodies (from insecticides, drugs, smoking and the like).

Other Uses of Pantothenic Acid

There are other essential functions of pantothenic acid. Several studies indicate that when consumed in the form calcium pantothenate, this vitamin can dramatically improve the levels of stiffness and pain in sufferers with rheumatoid arthritis. Many doctors have reported great success for treating rheumatoid arthritis when using this supplement with their patients.

Additionally, when pantothenic acid is taken in pantethine form, it has a very beneficial effect in reducing levels of triglycerides and cholesterol. Researchers think this may be because of its ability to increase the body's use of fat as a fuel source.

Thiamin (Vitamin B1)

To better understand what thiamin does in the body, consider the word that describes thiamin deficiency: beriberi. This east-Asian word means, literally, "I can't, I can't." And people suffering from beriberi can't do a lot. They are weak, fatigued, and without appetite. They may have numb or burning feet, cramps, and often, mental confusion.

This sets up one of most remarkable "miracles" of modern medicine. A beriberi patient, even at the brink of death, suffering from edema (a sort of internal "flooding" of the body by fluids), breathless and completely incapacitated, can receive a thiamin injection and be on his feet within a couple hours, completely (or nearly completely) recovered.

Thiamin and Brain Function

Thiamin's ability to enhance the body's energy production has ramifications for the brain as well. If thiamin intake is dramatically reduced, the brain is severely limited in its ability to use glucose (blood sugar). Because the brain has a very difficult time using energy sources other than glucose (unlike other body parts, which can switch to other types of fuels if necessary), its functioning slows. This creates a state of impaired mental function.

B VITAMIN COMPLEX FAST FACTS

Possible Benefits: The benefits are wide reaching, from relief of depression and cancer prevention to reduction of heart disease risk and premenstrual symptoms. Additionally, all the B vitamins are involved in dozens of vital body processes that help the body maintain proper functioning.

Special Instructions: Because most of the B vitamins rely on each other for proper function, take B vitamins all together either as a B-complex supplement or as part of a multivitamin/mineral supplement. Only take them individually if you know for sure that you are deficient or if you have a specific disorder that could require therapeutic doses. Always consult with a qualified health care provider before beginning any such therapy.

Product Forms: B vitamins are found together in B-complex supplements or as part of daily multivitamin supplements. Specific B vitamins are also sold individually.

Thiamin is also pertinent for the synthesis of critical neurotransmitters in the brain, including acetylcholine, which is involved in memory and performance. This is another way thiamin deficiency can negatively affect the brain. There are a number of studies showing that supplementing with thiamin clearly benefits those taking it, by improving memory and enhancing feelings of mental clarity and energy.

Niacin (Vitamin B3)

Niacin's discovery came about almost single-handedly because of the efforts to cure pellagra, a condition marked by diarrhea, dementia and a dark flaking of the skin. In the early 1900s, it was discovered that niacin was not present in corn, which by that time had become a principal food staple in North America and many parts of Europe. Pellagra reached epidemic proportions in the southeastern U.S., due to a large dependence on corn grits as a diet staple. In 1915, pellagra killed ten thousand people, and between 1917 and 1918, over two hundred thousand were inflicted with the disease.

Soon it was discovered that pellagra was a diseased caused by a deficiency, not an infectious agent, and subsequently corn was soon pinpointed as a primary cause because of its lack of niacin content. Today, nearly everyone gets enough niacin. Eggs, meat, poultry and fish are rich in this B vitamin, thus making pellagra largely a thing of the past.

Niacin: All-Around Booster

As is the case with most other B vitamins, niacin is used in a wide variety of body processes, including that of aiding the many enzymes that keep our bodies functioning. Niacin is a major player in the process of breaking down ingested foods into the forms of energy that our cells can either use immediately or store for later use. The enzymes that depend on niacin "package" this energy and release it in a proper and timely fashion. The same enzymes that depend on niacin for proper operating also assist in the handling of fat and cholesterol and the creation of other biochemicals, including hormones.

Heart Helper

There is research showing that relatively large doses of nicotinic acid and inositol hexaniacinate (both forms of niacin) do a good job of reducing cholesterol, possibly by improving liver function, and of raising the HDL cholesterol (the beneficial kind). In fact, many experts consider these two vitamin forms to be more effective at raising HDL levels than just about any synthetic drug available. One note of caution here. If you are considering using supplemental niacin for lowering cholesterol/raising HDL levels, it would be wise to have your program supervised by a knowledgeable health professional, as high doses have been linked to possible liver problems.

Biotin

Similar to its B vitamin cousins, biotin is necessary for a variety of vital body processes. It plays an important role in metabolism by acting as a coenzyme that helps transport carbon dioxide from compound to compound. It also helps convert various chemically important substances for processes such as protein synthesis, the formation of long-chain fatty acids, and the Krebs cycle, which is the basic process that releases energy from food.

Luckily, most people never become deficient in biotin. However, there are some individuals that suffer from absorption problems, especially those with Crohn's disease, that could become deficient. Some infants also suffer from a genetic problem that limits their ability to absorb biotin.

The thing for which biotin may be most well-known is its role in strengthening fingernails and hair. This is because it helps the body utilize certain fatty acids to create keratin, the protein substance that largely comprises nails and hair.

Another area that biotin supplementation could be of help in is with diabetes. Several studies show that taking extra biotin can enhance the performance of insulin, the hormone crucial for blood sugar utilization. Biotin supplements have also been shown to increase the activity of the enzyme used by the liver to begin utilizing blood sugar. One study focusing on individuals with type 1 diabetes found significant improvements in blood sugar control.

Another testing type 2 diabetics found that blood sugar levels fell approximately 50 percent after only one month. Another study indicates that biotin supplementation could be very helpful in treating severe diabetic nerve disease.

Riboflavin (Vitamin B2)

If you take a multivitamin or B-complex vitamin pill, you may notice that soon after taking it, your urine takes on a yellow-green glow. This is due to the riboflavin excess in the supplement. Now, riboflavin does much more than just produce psychedelic urine. It is a key player in the body's production of energy, just as many of its B vitamin cousins. In short, riboflavin aids in the process that produces ATP, the body's basic energy currency. ATP is used extensively throughout our bodies any time energy is needed—to move muscles, digest food, breathe, make protein, etc. If riboflavin is in short supply, we feel lethargic.

It also helps the body produce glutathione, which is a potent antioxidant that can protect us from cellular damage that can lead to cancer, heart disease and a myriad of other conditions. For instance, research has shown that riboflavin deficiencies lead to the development of cataracts. This is because glutathione helps protect the eyes against cellular damage caused by sunlight and other factors.

Another area for which riboflavin may be helpful is migraine headaches. Researchers have shown that there can be a significant reduction of severity and frequency of migraine headaches with the addition of daily riboflavin supplements; enough of a reduction, in fact, that the supplement's effects were then compared to standard migraine drugs.

The Bottom Line

As you can see, the B vitamins are vitally important for good health. A deficiency of any of them can create a domino effect resulting in various health problems. The B vitamins are crucial to proper body functioning, from creating and maintaining energy production, to assisting enzymes in their myriad of functions, to assisting in the creation of red blood cells. Deficiencies of the eight B vitamins are linked to a host of ailments, ranging from heart disease to dementia to cancer. While they are usually found in adequate amounts in a well-rounded diet, there is ample research suggesting that many individuals do not have such a diet; thus, taking a B-vitamin complex supplement could help treat and prevent a wide variety of diseases and promote overall health.

5

Echinacea

MOST OF US are aware that our immune systems are made up of several different organs and cells, all of which have different and specialized assignments in defending the body against invaders. There are white blood cells, natural killer cells, macrophages and other defense cells that roam the body on a special mission—identifying, ingesting and destroying specific pathogens, such as viruses, bacteria and fungi. This process is called phagocytosis (after the word *phagocyte*, which is an umbrella term for the cells that finish up the dirty work of killing harmful substances), and if your immune system is functioning optimally, few foreign agents can survive in the body.

However, most of us know that today's lifestyle leads more and more of us to a declined state of health, and therefore, depressed immunity. But one herbal agent in particular—echinacea—can help rev up your immune

FROM AMERICA TO GERMANY ...
... AND BACK AGAIN

One intriguing historical note regarding echinacea surrounds its use by Native Americans and early European-Americans until the beginning of the twentieth century. Many historical accounts of Native Americans and how they dealt with disease detail how the echinacea plant was used for a variety of problems, including snakebite, wounds and infections.

However, just like many of the natural remedies that were prevalent, echinacea fell out of favor with the American public with the emergence of synthetic pharmaceuticals. However, interest on part of European countries continued strong. In fact, one German company began to import echinacea seeds from North America with the intent of conducting research on it. Over the next fifty years or so, dozens of studies were conducted, mainly using products created from the Echinacea purpurea species.

The immense popularity of echinacea in Germany and other European countries speaks something of its efficacy. It is estimated that in 1994, there were more than three hundred echinacea products on the German market, and German doctors issued more than two and a half million prescriptions for this herb alone.

Now, because of widespread use in Germany, Britain

and other countries, echinacea has once again become extremely popular in the United States. In fact, it is one of the top-selling herbal products among a large boom in natural remedies.

function by enhancing the ability of your immune cells to fight foreign agents and also by killing a few of those agents itself.

Germ Warfare: In the Trenches

There are a number of herbs that are immunostimulants—agents that stimulate your body's immune defenses to fight off illness and infection. Echinacea is one of the best known of these natural agents and one with the most science to support it. In fact, there have been literally hundreds of studies done on the various species of echinacea, with most of this coming in the last fifty years.

How does echinacea work? Essentially, it speeds up immune function, increasing the number of white blood cells to hunt down foreign agents and speeding up the entire process of phagocytosis. So, in this way it is a classic stimulator of the immune system, giving impetus to the body's own defense mechanisms to work harder and enhancing their capabilities.

This is especially important when you consider illness like the flu or the common cold. Studies show that taking echinacea at the very onset of a cold or flu can both stop the progression of the infection and shorten the duration and lessen the severity of the symptoms.

There are other ways that echinacea works to defend your body against unwanted invaders. First, some research indicates that it directly seeks and kills certain viruses. This means that it has a direct deadly effect on the germ and doesn't rely on the body's immunity cells to do the work. Additionally, echinacea seems to prevent the action of an enzyme called hyaluronidase. When you're sick, this enzyme breaks down the walls of healthy cells, thereby allowing the infectious agents to take them over. But echinacea can interfere with the activity of hyaluronidase, thus permitting the body to keep healthy cells . . . well . . . healthy. How echinacea actually interferes with the enzyme isn't quite clear. Some researchers actually think that it doesn't really interfere with the enzyme at all, but rather fortifies the cell wall so the enzyme has a more difficult time breaking it down. Either way, the consensus is that the effects of hyaluronidase enzyme are weakened when in the presence of echinacea.

In addition to being taken internally for stimulation of the immune system, echinacea can also be used topically for wounds, infections, inflammation and other skin problems. Echinacea has antifungal and antibacterial properties that allow topical wounds and internal infections, such as the often-difficult candida, to heal more quickly.

But Does It Really Work? What the Studies Say

So much has been written regarding echinacea and its health benefits that it may take some time before the entire truth can be told. However, while some experts believe that more human studies are needed to definitively recommend the herb as a viable medicine, the majority of health experts at least agree that echinacea does offer some therapeutic firepower, with most of that centered in its ability to stimulate the immune system.

Regarding human studies, most of them have involved small groups and were not well designed, at least by Western scientific/medical standards (meaning they were not randomized, placebo-controlled, or double-blind studies). Also, the bulk of the studies performed in Germany involved injectable formulas not available here in the U.S., and many of the studies did not test echinacea by itself, thereby making it more difficult to attribute favorable results to echinacea.

Still, significant therapeutic potential has been documented in both test-tube and animal studies for the upper parts of *E. purpurea* and the roots of other echinacea species. Some of these studies indicate that the extracts of the plant fight certain viruses, including influenza and herpes. These studies showed that cells immersed in echinacea extracts could defend themselves much better from the flu and herpes viruses than could cells not exposed to echinacea. And, as discussed earlier, many studies at least indicate that echinacea can indeed kick-start the immune system to function better and faster.

German health authorities specifically endorse the aforementioned parts of the various echinacea species for recurring respiratory and urinary tract infections. Findings also confirm the value of echinacea in treating superficial, poorly healing cuts, scrapes, cold sores and psoriasis lesions.

ECHINACEA FAST FACTS

Scientific Names: Echinacea purpurea, Echinacea angustifolia, Echinacea pallida

Common Names: American coneflower, purple coneflower, black sampson, black susan, Kansas snake root

Possible Benefits: Depressed immune function, common infections, chronic fatigue syndrome, common cold, bronchitis, ear infections, flu, cystitis, laryngitis, diverticulitis, celiac disease

Special Instructions: Begin use at first sign of cold, flu or other infection. Many experts warn that continual, long-term use can lessen its effectiveness. Also, people with autoimmune disorders should probably not use echinacea, nor should those who are allergic to plants in the daisy family, such as chamomile and marigold.

What about the safety and any side effects of using echinacea? No significant side effects have been reported. And this is saying something due to the fact that literally hundreds of thousands of people use echinacea every year. The only real safety recommendation is for those individuals suffering from autoimmune disorders, such as lupus, or severe systemic diseases such as multiple sclerosis, tuberculosis or AIDS.

The Bottom Line

There is little doubt that echinacea can offer a safe and powerful boost to your immune function. Because so much of our health depends on the workings of an effective immune system, this makes echinacea quite valuable indeed.

At the onset of a cold, flu or other infection, you may want to increase your initial amounts to give your immune system a jumpstart, especially in the first twenty-four hours or so of the illness. This revved-up effect, however, is usually fairly short lived. As mentioned earlier, the longer echinacea is used, the less effective it appears to be. Consequently, you'll want to use it only when you feel sickness approaching and not on a continual basis. So, if everyone at the office is sick, or your kids come home from school with signs of the flu, the bottom line is—take it.

6

Probiotics: Beneficial Bacteria

WHEN WE HEAR the word "bacteria," we usually think of something harmful or unsanitary. Perhaps images of dirty bathrooms, spoiled food or scrapes from rusty nails come to mind. Well, unknown to many people is the fact that many of the types of bacteria that occupy our bodies (and environment) are actually good for us. Constantly performing good work in our intestinal tract and elsewhere are literally hundreds of species of microscopic bacteria that promote healthy digestion, produce needed vitamins, fight infection, and enhance immune function, among other functions. *Lactobacillus acidophilus* (often just called "acidophilus") and *Bifidobacterium bifidum* are a few of the stars of these "probiotics," or beneficial bacteria.

We are not born with a ready-made supply of these beneficial bacteria, but we begin acquiring them soon after birth. An infant's mother contributes greatly to the growth of bacteria through her breast milk. As the infant grows and consumes other types of food, additional bacteria—both good and bad—begin to colonize throughout the body. As we get older, it is imperative that we maintain optimal levels of good bacteria in order to keep the bad varieties in check, and thereby prevent the onset of a variety of diseases.

Intestinal Bacteria: Friend or Foe?

There are more than four hundred different species of bacteria and more than one hundred trillion separate organisms—of which relatively few are beneficial—that inhabit the intestinal tract. Thus it is imperative that friendly bacteria are maintained at optimal levels. And what makes a particular bacteria friendly? Acidophilus, bifidobacterium and other bacteria are considered friendly or beneficial because they help produce vital nutrients such as B vitamins, they produce enzymes necessary to for top-notch digestion, they promote improved immune function, and they "stake out" their own territory, thereby preventing harmful bacteria, fungi and yeast from multiplying and creating a hazardous health condition.

Why might you need to take a probiotic supplement? For starters, many factors can deplete beneficial bacteria levels, including poor diet, stress, disease, high levels of toxins, too much sugar/refined carbohydrates, and alcohol/tobacco use. As soon as the presence of the good guys diminishes, the bad guys naturally move in to take their place. If this cycle continues for long, the harmful bacteria will eventually multiply to the point that they have "take over" the gut, contributing to many and serious health conditions.

Antibiotics: No Longer the Answer

When it comes to enemies of our body's friendly bacteria, one of the most menacing may be something that is supposed to be helpful—antibiotics. While it is true that these prescription drugs can indeed wipe out dangerous bacteria, they wipe out the beneficial ones as well. Improper use of antibiotics sets the stage for secondary infections, and eventually, resistance to the drug by the original invading bacteria.

For instance, if an antibiotic is working in the vaginal area, the result can be very counterproductive. Vaginal yeast is held in check by acidophilus and other beneficial bacteria, and once that barrier is removed by the antibiotic, the yeast can multiply and spread quickly, causing what is otherwise known as a yeast infection. Chronic yeast infections are an increasingly common health complaint among women and can lead to more serious health conditions.

This is where probiotics can provide some definite answers—restoring levels of friendly flora to keep the bad ones in check. It's true that while acute yeast infections can be treated with relatively safe over-the-counter medications, these remedies don't offer anything in the way of long-term solutions to chronic infections. Probiotic sup-

WHICH BACTERIA ARE BEST?

As mentioned earlier, there are literally hundreds of different species of bacteria that inhabit the body, yet only a handful are helpful. The following overview provides a look at the probiotics that offer you the most punch for great health.

Lactobacillus acidophilus: Often just called acidophilus, the genus/species *L. acidophilus* actually has approximately two hundred strains, of which the most beneficial are the NAS and DDS-1 strains. Both of these are highly recommended as being the most effective against the most pathogens, including *Bacilus subtilis*, *Serratia marcescens*, *Proteus vulgaris*, *Pseudomonas fluorescens*, *Pseudomonas aeruginosa*, *Escherichia coli*, *Sarcina lutea*, *Staphylococcus aureus*, and *Streptococcus lactis*. They have also been shown to inhibit fungal growth, relieve chronic states of constipation and diarrhea, produce the necessary digestive enzyme lactase, and improve the absorption of nutrients (especially calcium).

Bifidobacterium bifidum: This important strain of probiotic, which normally inhabits the large intestine of adults, is known as a "bully" among beneficial bacteria because of its tendency to become very aggressive with pathogenic invaders. This strain also inhibits the bacteria responsible for turning nitrates into cancer-causing nitrites and for aiding in the proper production of B vitamins. Interestingly, bifidobacterium may work better for those people who don't experience benefit from *L. acidophilus*. And many experts consider it to be preferable to acidophilus for children and adults with liver disorders.

There is also a growing body of research on the *B. bifidum* Malyoth "superstrain" that indicates it has widespread health benefits, including helping in the detoxification of the liver, preventing malabsorption of nutrients and B-vitamin deficiencies, regulating the production of waste, and preventing diarrhea, constipation and the onset of chronic immune suppression.

Lactobacillus bulgaricus: This helpful bacteria is a sort of transient that is most helpful in the colonizing of other probiotics. One of the most notable strains of *L. bulgaricus*—LB-51—has received high praise for its ability to correct a variety of digestive problems. But it can do more than that. LB-51 has shown itself to be a powerful antibiotic agent that can work against specific harmful bacteria and stimulate immune response. Research also indicates that because of its ability to maintain a clean intestinal tract, waste disposal is maximized and related problems (constipation, diarrhea, etc.) are alleviated.

> ***Lactobacillus GG (LGG):*** A relative newcomer to the probiotic scene, *LGG* has been available in supplement form in this country only since 1998. Many experts believe that it is superior to *L. acidophilus* in its ability to fight gastrointestinal disorders. In fact, there is such a huge body of research on *LGG*'s beneficial attributes that it is scientifically more supported than acidophilus or other probiotics. One reason may be that it is derived from a sterile form of the bacteria that grows in the human intestine, whereas acidophilus comes from a dairy strain. This may better equip *LGG* to survive in the gastrointestinal and vaginal tracts than acidophilus and the other friendly probiotic strains.

plements, on the other hand, can provide the long-term answer by helping to reestablish the colonies of bifidobacterium, acidophilus and other beneficial bacteria and maintain a proper and healthy balance in the vaginal and intestinal systems.

The Probiotic Problem: Ensuring Live Cells

When considering a probiotic supplement, you may be faced with the dilemma of choosing between dozens of different products. One of the most important things to remember is that these bacteria are live organisms, and for them to be of help, they must be living when you ingest them. The following guidelines will aid you in making sure you're getting the highest-quality product.

- Some experts caution against taking products that have mixed strains of probiotics, especially if they don't list the counts of each individual bacteria. In this case, you may not get enough of the bacteria that you want. Good advice would be to purchase different products that each contain one specific probiotic strain, then take them intermittently.

- Most experts recommend looking for a count of at least one billion organisms per capsule, or two billion organisms per teaspoon. Some products offer even higher counts.

- Probiotics are available in several different forms, including powder, capsule, tablet, wafer and liquids. Many experts recommend the powder form as being best, but many also indicate that the capsule form, especially an enteric-coated capsule, may be desirable since it can pass through the stomach into the intestinal tract before releasing the bacteria. Some literature discourages the use of liquid probiotics, as they can lose their potency fairly quickly.

- Ensure that your product has a guaranteed expiration date. If it doesn't, don't buy it. Also, beware of products that states something like "at the time of manufacture" or "at the time of shipment." Who knows how long after those dates you will actually buy the product!

- Avoid products that indicate they have undergone a "centrifuge" or "ultrafiltration" process. These processes can break down the bacteria, rendering them less effective or even useless. They also artificially inflate the bacterial count (by including damaged/partial organisms in the count).

- Take your probiotic on an empty stomach first thing in the morning, and then close to meal times throughout the day. Also, some experts recommend taking it with filtered, lukewarm water (as tap water may contain chlorine, which will kill bacteria, and cold water can have a debilitating effect on bacteria as well).

- Keep your probiotics in a cool, dry place, with the lid kept on tight. The refrigerator is a great place to keep it (though be careful it doesn't freeze).

- If you're having a tough time deciding what to get, let the price be your guide. While it is no guarantee, the cheaper products generally indicate an inferior product.

- If you are taking an antibiotic, some experts recommend doubling or even tripling your normal probiotic dose during and up to three weeks after finishing your antibiotic treatment. However, make sure to not take them simultaneously (as the probiotic will be killed by the antibiotic). Take the probiotic a minimum of two hours after taking your antibiotic.

PROBIOTIC FAST FACTS

Popular Strains: Lactobacillus acidophilus, Lactobacillus bulgaricus, Bifidobacterium bifidum, Lactobacillus GG

Possible Benefits: Chronic yeast infections (in vagina and elsewhere), urinary tract infections, lactose intolerance, diarrhea, constipation, faltering immune function, irritable bowel syndrome, lupus, fibromyalgia, high cholesterol, indigestion, malabsorption of nutrients, bloating, gas, osteoporosis, production of B vitamins, production of digestive enzymes

Dietary Sources: Fermented milk products, including yogurt and kefir

Possible Side Effects: Overall, supplementing with probiotic products is extremely safe. However, if you suffer from a severe gastrointestinal problem, it would be wise to consult with you healthcare provider before starting a regimen of probiotic supplements. Also, some reports indicate that exceeding ten billion viable organisms daily may cause mild gastrointestinal distress.

The Bottom Line

The literal mountain of research on friendly bacteria indicates that they can have a tremendous impact on our health. We know they are vital to the health of our digestive and gastrointestinal tracts. They ward off dangerous pathogens, including harmful bacteria, fungus and yeast such as *Candida albicans*. Probiotics also improve the production of vital nutrients, such as B vitamins, as well as the production of digestive enzymes. They discourage infections of the vagina and urinary tract, prevent diarrhea and constipation, alleviate various gastrointestinal ills, lower high cholesterol and can even relieve symptoms of lupus and fibromyalgia. In other words, supplementing with these friendly bacteria can produce wide-reaching benefits for you and your health.

7

Astragalus

ALTHOUGH ONLY RECENTLY INTRODUCED into Western culture, astragalus has been valued in China as a tonic and potent medicinal agent for more than two thousand years. Traditional healers there regard it as one of the premier immune-enhancing herbal medicines that also has adaptogenic properties. An adaptogen is something that helps the body return to normal functioning. For instance, an adaptogen that is helpful to restore normal blood pressure will both lower high blood pressure and raise low blood pressure. Traditional Chinese healers also believe astragalus is a warming tonic for increased resistance to cold. They also believe it can help the body replenish its vital energy, called *chi*. Chinese doctors usually mix astragalus with other herbs, depending on a person's complaint. Their overall focus is to "tone" the body and help it adapt to the stressors affecting it.

From a Western perspective, astragalus is considered an immune-enhancing botanical agent, capable of improving the body's response to invading pathogens, including bacteria, viruses, and other toxins, and aid the body in faster recovery of various conditions, including cancer. Moreover, there is evidence that it can provide protection from a variety of health problems, including the common cold and flu (and other common infections), secondary infections resulting from chemotherapy/radiation therapy, diabetes, fibromyalgia, chronic fatigue syndrome, stomach ulcers, chronic diarrhea, viral heart damage, high blood pressure, burns, wounds and abscesses.

Defending the Body

For centuries, astragalus has been employed in fu-zheng therapy, a treatment used by traditional Chinese healers to bolster the immune system. In attempting to improve the immune function of their patients, these practitioners have even begun to use fu-zheng therapy to help with cancer patients. They use astragalus to boost immune function before, during and after radiation or chemotherapy treatments.

When cancer progresses in the body, your immune system naturally becomes weakened. In the advanced stages of the disease, or after treatments of chemotherapy or radiation therapy, your immune system can become literally devastated. Because of this, any number of opportunistic infections, such as colds or flu, can overcome the weak-

> **ASTRAGALUS AND BONE MARROW**
>
> One way that astragalus appears to stimulate the immune system is by influencing bone marrow, which is where many of our immune cells are manufactured. Polysaccharides (which are healthy sugars) seem to stimulate white blood cell production and increase the activity of killer T cells, which are one of the body's principal defenders against invading pathogens.
>
> Additionally, astragalus increases the production of another immune substance, interferon, a natural protein that sticks to the surfaces of cells. In simple terms, it helps make your cells more thick skinned so viruses have a difficult time invading.

ened immune defenses and turn into a very serious, even deadly, infection.

The effectiveness of astragalus in a fu-zheng treatment was examined in a study involving nineteen cancer patients at the M.D. Anderson Cancer Center in Houston. These patients were given a special astragalus extract, and doctors found that the therapy restored immune functioning in the majority of the patients, even to resemble the immune systems of normal people in some cases. The study's authors had very positive words for the astragalus extract, concluding that it did represent a potentially powerful immune stimulant.

Other intriguing studies indicate that astragalus can indeed stimulate the immune system. One study revealed that astragalus may act as an immune stimulant for AIDS patients; the same study indicates that the herb could inhibit immune system suppression resulting from chemotherapy.

ASTRAGALUS FAST FACTS

Scientific Name: Astragalus membranaceus; also known as huang qi in Chinese medicine.

Possible Benefits: Suppressed immunity due to disease, including cancer; high stress levels; chronic fatigue syndrome; common infections, including colds and flu; fibromyalgia; respiratory disease; and chronic, lingering diarrhea.

Safety Issues: Astragalus is generally regarded as safe. Its toxicity appears to be very low, considering that it has been used for centuries in various cultures. Also findings of modern research show little danger in using astragalus.

Origin: Medicinal species grows only in Asia.

Heart Health and Other Benefits of Astragalus

Astragalus appears to benefit the body in several other ways. One way in particular is the protection of the heart. According to several studies, the herb appears to positively affect damaged heart tissue. One study showed that heart attack victims treated with the herb suffered less angina (chest pain) and experienced more improvement in EKG readings and other measurements than subjects given standard heart medications, such as nifedipine. Another study found that the herb had a tonic effect on the hearts of patients hospitalized with heart attacks over a four-week span, compared with patients not given the herbal preparation.

Several other studies have shown that astragalus fights the effects of the Coxsackie B virus, which can cause scarring, inflammation, and other forms of heart damage. Authors of these studies have indicated that the herb may represent a favorable option in treating individuals with heart problems stemming from infection of the Coxsackie B virus.

In addition to improving the health of the heart, astragalus may offer benefits in other areas. Research has uncovered possible uses of astragalus for inflammation, sub-par memory and learning performance, low stamina, hepatitis-related liver damage, erratic blood sugar levels, and for use as a diuretic for favorable output of urine.

The Bottom Line

In today's world it is becoming more difficult to achieve a healthy lifestyle—it is necessary to utilize outside help to both treat and prevent disease. Because of modern research and its use over thousands of years in various cultures, astragalus offers a wide variety of benefits, especially that of improving immune function. Of course, astragalus can benefit you in many other ways, from fighting heart disease to battling cancer to relieving chronic diarrhea. So, if you could only take one nutritional supplement, astragalus would certainly be a worthy choice.

8

Glyconutrients: Healthy Sugars

THOUGHT YOU'D NEVER SEE the day when you heard "sugar" could be good for you? Well that day is here. The notion that different sugars, otherwise called glyconutrients, offer many different health benefits is quickly becoming widely accepted. From immunity enhancement to chronic fatigue syndrome, glyconutrients are demonstrating potent health-promoting abilities.

So, what are glyconutrients? In simple terms, "glyco" essentially means "sweet." Thus, a glyconutrient is a biochemical that is partially made up of a sugar molecule. The prefix "glyco" can be placed at the front of a fat, protein or any other molecule, thereby suggesting that a sugar is attached to that molecule. The generic version of a sugar substance is called a "glycoform."

Can It Really Be Good for Me?

As mentioned previously, most of us grew up with the idea that sugar wasn't very good for us. And until recently, that idea was widely supported within the scientific community. Sucrose is the "sweet" sugar that we are most familiar with, but it also happens to be the worst for our health. In fact, sucrose is dangerously overused in America. The average yearly consumption of refined white sugar in this country has rocketed from approximately six pounds at the turn of the century to over 150 pounds today. Refined sucrose is nothing but empty calories and offers nothing in the way of any nutritional value. However, there are a number of other sugars that play a pivotal role in our good health, providing benefits such as improved immune function, proper regulation of blood sugar and inflammatory conditions, fighting arthritis, and cancer prevention.

Essential Sugars: Immune Boosters Extraordinaire

Our modern lifestyles are making it more difficult for many of us to maintain a healthy immune system. Poor dietary and exercise habits, toxic environments, high levels of stress, and the overuse of antibiotics and other synthetic drugs all have an adverse effect on our immunity. Yet a strong immune system is the cornerstone to optimal health.

When discussing the immune system, it is important to remember that all diseases eventually are the result of malfunction at the cellular level. A healthy body is made up of healthy organs, which are comprised of healthy tissues made up of healthy cells. In essence, if our individual cells—the building blocks of the body—aren't healthy or are malfunctioning, then the domino effect of this on body tissues, organs or whole systems leads to some sort of diseased state.

Breakdowns in cellular communication are an example of cellular malfunction. If the communication between cells is impaired, then all sorts of potential problems may result. For instance, a healthy cell could be misidentified as a foreign body, thereby triggering the immune system to attack it. This could ultimately lead to an autoimmune response (such as what we see in those people with lupus, fibromyalgia and rheumatoid arthritis). Also, communication failures may lead to overlooked cancerous cells by the various immune responses, resulting in cancer.

That's where glyconutrients come in. Earlier, we mentioned that certain essential glyconutrients can improve cellular communication and function. In short, increased consumption of these essential sugars (whether through the diet or through supplements) can help correct an overactive immune system (evident in autoimmune diseases), stimulate an underactive immune system, and keep our various immune responses in optimal shape for overall disease prevention.

So, how do these sugars help keep the immune system

SUGAR, SUGAR EVERYWHERE

Everyone has heard of sucrose, but here are a few other sugar names that you might want to become a bit more familiar with, as well as their health benefits:

Glucose: This sugar is quite abundant in our diets and is in fact overconsumed. It's converted from food sources such as potatoes, rice and other sugary and starchy foods.

Fucose: This saccharide is not readily available in food. However, it is abundant in breast milk (thus it plays a vital role in helping develop the first immune responses of a nursing infant), as well as medicinal mushrooms such as maitake. Fucose has been the focus of many scientific studies targeting its immune-enhancing abilities.

Galactose: This sugar is commonly found in most diets, with its primary sources being dairy foods (converted from milk sugar, called lactose).

Mannose: This is another powerful health-promoting glyconutrient. It is vital to proper cellular function and can positively affect the body's immune response against pathogens. Additionally, there is research that suggests mannose may have anti-inflammatory and blood sugar-lowering capabilities.

Xylose: Not available in most diets, xylose is commonly used to help sweeten sugarless gum. (It is interesting to note that although it has a sweet taste, it does not adversely affect the enamel of the tooth.) Like other essential saccharides, xylose helps fights microbial invaders such as fungus and bacteria and may also fight cancer. It has been featured in allergy nasal spray products due to its ability to discourage the binding of allergens to mucous membranes.

N-acetyl-galactosamine: Not readily available in our diet, this essential sugar plays an important role in promoting proper function of and communication between cells. In addition, there is mounting evidence that it can help fight the growth of some cancers.

N-acetyl-glucosamine: This glyconutrient can be very helpful for the proper maintenance of our joints, and can reverse (or prevent) cartilage and joint damage/inflammation. The popular supplement glucosamine, which is now widely recognized for its abilities to fight arthritic conditions, is derived from n-acetyl-glucosamine.

N-acetyl-neuramic acid: Like other essential saccharides, this is also abundantly found in breast milk and can have a significantly healthy effect on the nervous

> system from the time a fetus begins growing. N-acetyl-neuramic acid also possesses the ability to stimulate immune function.
>
> *Arabinogalactan:* This sugar has demonstrated a wide variety of health-promoting effects, including the ability to fight specific cancers, hepatitis B and C, chronic fatigue and infections.

functioning exceptionally? Here are a few ways. They can:

- stimulate T-cell activity only when foreign antigens are present.
- significantly increase the counts of natural killer cells and macrophages.
- demonstrate antioxidant capabilities, thereby fighting the effects of free radicals and reducing stress on the body and its immune defenses.
- optimize the communication between cells, which is crucial for normal immune function.
- aid in the reduction of inflammation.

Autoimmune Disorders and Glyconutrients

There are numerous studies linking essential-sugar deficiencies to the onset of various autoimmune diseases, which are typically characterized by the body's own immune cells (such as killer cells, T cells and the like) attacking healthy and otherwise friendly cells. This can cause inflammation, pain, soreness and other effects that are often debilitating to the sufferer. Below is a brief discussion of how a lack or malfunction of glyconutrients can lead to the development of an autoimmune response in some of today's most prominent autoimmune conditions:

Lupus: Deficiencies of mannose-binding proteins have been linked to lupus, an autoimmune condition that is often very serious. A 1996 study published in *Arthritis and Rheumatism* concluded that inadequate levels of these proteins can indeed raise one's risk of developing lupus. This reiterates the idea that because optimal cellular communication is necessary to maintain a healthy immune system (and thereby avoid autoimmune responses), supplementation with glyconutrients should be a consideration.

Rheumatoid Arthritis: This form of arthritis is characterized by inflammation and pain in the joints due to the body's own defense cells attacking healthy cells in the joint areas. Interestingly, there are several studies showing that low levels of the saccharide, fucose, are linked to even the most severe forms of rheumatism. Doris Lefkowitz, Ph.D., has studied the disease intensively and concluded that in addition to fucose, another essential sugar, galactose, is present only in minimal levels of many individuals suffering from rheumatoid arthritis. Additionally, she cites abnormal cell communications as a reason for continued immune response dysfunction.

It is noteworthy to consider that another glyconutrient, n-acetyl-glucosamine, can be very helpful in reducing swelling in joints and surrounding areas and to help regenerate cartilage tissue.

Dermatomyositis: This arthritis-like disease is characterized by the presence of sugars whose structural makeups have been altered after a parasitic infection, thereby rendering them useless and possibly even dangerous. Remember that cellular communications are compromised whenever the sugar component of a molecule is missing or damaged. This leads to the breakdown of communication between immune cells and other healthy cells, and can ultimately lead to the body's own healthy cells being attacked by friendly immunity cells. Dermatomyositis shows the same profile as several other autoimmune disorders—a lack of essential sugars, abnormalities in their structures or an inability to absorb and utilize them.

Can Glyconutrients Beat Cancer?

We all are familiar with cancer and its deadly statistics. The fact is that approximately one in every three Americans will develop some form of cancer in their lifetime. All of us, however, can take steps to become one of the "other two" who don't develop cancer.

The best step is to improve our immune function. Those persons with suppressed immune systems have the greatest risk of developing cancer.

The immune system fights and destroys cancer cells every day. And as we have already discussed, a key aspect of the immune system is its ability to communicate effectively between cells to identify those that are friendly and those that aren't. The presence of adequate levels of the different essential sugars helps to achieve that communication.

There is a growing body of research that points to deficiencies of and abnormalities in different saccharides being intimately linked to cancer, including stomach, colon and breast cancer. For instance, research published in *Cancer Research* showed that deformed or absent sugars have been specifically linked to the formation of stomach cancer. Most of the known polysaccharides, or glyconutrients, have been shown to either fight cancer directly or to stimulate the immune system in such a way as to specifically fight cancer.

Glyconutrients and Other Health Conditions

Chronic Fatigue Syndrome: Though the exact causes of this disease still are not understood, it is often characterized by the presence of autoimmune dysfunction. In one recent study involving chronic fatigue patients, the addition of supplemental polysaccharides increased levels of

GLYCONUTRIENT FAST FACTS

Natural Sources: There are various foods and other natural sources of glyconutrients, including many that have been used specifically as health-promoting agents.

- **Breast milk** contains at least five essential sugars, which strongly suggests that the body requires these and other saccharides to develop correctly.
- **Astragalus**, which is widely recognized as a premiere immune stimulator, contains several sugars, including fucose, xylose, arabinose and galactose.
- **Aloe vera**, which is also known for various health-promoting properties, contains several essential saccharides.
- **Maitake and shiitake mushrooms**, which have been used for thousands of years in Asian cultures, contain high levels of beta-glucans, which are high in mannose and other sugars and have been shown to optimize immune function in various ways.
- **Pectin**, widely known for its use in making jellies, jams and the like, provides a form of fiber that can lower cholesterol and contains several essential sugars. It is thought that a high-fruit diet is helpful in preventing cancer due in part due to its saccharide and pectin content.
- **The sap of the larch tree** contains the saccharide ara-

binogalactan, which has been shown to help battle cancerous tumors, fight chronic fatigue syndrome, increase levels of beneficial intestinal bacteria, and fight hepatitis B and C viruses.

Product Availability: Though they are fairly new to consumer markets, glyconutrient products are becoming more widely available and can be found in health food stores and through health product distributors. While some products contain only a single glyconutrient, most contain an assortment of sugars (which we recommend since the body is generally lacking in more than one). Glyconutritionals may be called "sugars," "essential sugars," "essential saccharides," "polysaccharides" or something with the root "glyco" on the front (i.e. "glyconutrients," "glyconutritionals," etc.). They are currently available as extracts, powders or freeze-dried capsules.

Possible Side Effects: As of this writing, there is no indication that properly supplementing with glyconutritional products is unsafe (though like any supplement, you should consult with your health care provider if you have questions or concerns regarding the supplement you are taking). However, the safety of these products for pregnant and/or nursing women has not been established.

natural killer cells, stopped premature cell death and increased other general indicators of improved immune function.

Candidiasis: This condition, which is characterized by the overgrowth of the yeast *Candida albicans*, can lead to other debilitating conditions. There is some promising research involving glyconutrients and candida, including one study published showing that the polysaccharide mannose quickens the destruction of yeast organisms. Also, researchers at the University of Kuwait found that the addition of the sugars mannose and N-acetyl-glucosamine was very effective in preventing the formation of yeast in the digestive tracts of mice.

Fibromyalgia: Like chronic fatigue syndrome, doctors and health experts do not understand what causes this disease, which is characterized by chronic muscle and tissue tenderness, fatigue, disruptive sleep patterns and various other symptoms. Some research points to low levels of serotonin as a culprit in fibromyalgia's development. Glyconutrients can have tremendous impact on the brain and its chemical production. In fact, recent research shows that when particular polysaccharides aren't properly interacting with certain brain chemicals, their uptake by surrounding cells is decreased. Also, a 2002 study showed that individuals with fibromyalgia who participated in a therapy that included the consumption of a combination of different supplements, among them essential sugars, experienced significant improvement in their symptoms.

There are numerous other health conditions where a lack of essential sugars may play a role. They include the following:

- urinary tract infections
- ulcers
- ADHD
- heart disease
- Alzheimer's and other dementia

The Bottom Line

Not all sugars are created equal. In fact, some sugars can be life savers. Glyconutrients are a great way to boost the immune system, especially for those under a lot of stress or otherwise at increased risk for illness and those suffering from chronic or acute disease, including autoimmune disorders and even cancer.

9

Beta Carotene and Vitamin A

CARROTS, SQUASH, CANTALOUPE, broccoli, kale, yellow peppers. They all contain beta carotene. Liver, milk, eggs. They all contain vitamin A.

At first glance, these two sources of nutrients seem to be quite distant. One is from the plant world, while the other is all animal. However, once the beta carotene from plant sources is absorbed in our bodies, it undergoes a transformation that makes it equal to the vitamin A found in animal sources. And the plant-source vitamin A provides all the health benefits of the animal-source version. Not only that, but once the transformation is complete and the body has all the vitamin A it needs, any excess beta carotene can be utilized for other needs.

As for the supplements that contain beta carotene and vitamin A, unfortunately, they're not equal. The problem

WHAT ARE BETA CAROTENE AND VITAMIN A?

Many people aren't really sure about the relationship of vitamin A and beta carotene, and rightly so. More than six hundred carotenoids (of which beta carotene is one) are found in nature, and about fifty of them have the potential to convert into one of several forms of vitamin A. The good thing is that if you eat a relatively balanced diet, you are bound to get the beta carotene and the vitamin A your body requires. Beta carotene can be found in oranges fruits and vegetables—like carrots and mangoes—and in green leafy vegetables—like broccoli, and vitamin A is found largely in animal products.

So what exactly is vitamin A? Here's the scoop: Vitamin A, like many other vitamins, is not actually one substance. There are several forms of vitamin A, each with slight differences in potency and action. The two main types are retinol and dehydroretinol. Then there are the carotenes, which are the precursors to vitamin A found in fruits and vegetables. Carotenes help us create vitamin A through several metabolic processes.

Of the most powerful carotenes, beta carotene is the heaviest hitter, providing about two-thirds of the vitamin A your body needs to survive. That's probably the sole reason it gets most of the attention when talk turns to vitamin A.

is that the pure form of vitamin A, called preformed vitamin A, can cause a number of nasty toxic effects if you take too much. Beta carotene is much more safe and can be taken in moderately large doses without any real threat of toxicity.

As for the history of vitamin A (and beta carotene), it is long and "colorful." Early remedies using vitamin A to treat night blindness (a condition in which your eyes lose their ability to adequately adjust to dim light) are cited in early Chinese texts. Later, in Greece, Hippocrates, the so-called father of modern medicine, utilized various liver preparations to treat the same condition, not knowing that liver is rich in vitamin A. Definitive findings on vitamin A came in 1913, when scientists operating independently discovered vitamin A in various fatty foods, mainly by showing that animals suffer vision problems when deprived of these foods. Later studies confirmed these findings, and thus proved Hippocrates right in his love of liver remedies for vision problems.

Years later, after other exciting findings, the true defining moment for vitamin A—and a defining moment for vitamins and nutrition in general—came when a Swiss scientist named Paul Karrar isolated the active substance in halibut liver oil. His work resulted in vitamin A being the first vitamin ever to have its chemical structure decoded. For this work, Karrar received the Nobel prize.

The Roles of Beta Carotene/Vitamin A

Vision

Vitamin A plays vital roles throughout the body. In our eyes, for instance, it helps maintain a crystal-clear outer window—the cornea. Without enough vitamin A, the cornea clouds over. At the back of the eye in the retina, vitamin A is part of the pigment that reacts chemically when struck by light. It assists in creating the nerve impulse the travels to the brain and ultimately creates a visual message. For this reason, vitamin A can help with the previously discussed condition of night blindness.

If your eyes don't have enough available vitamin A, they recover very slowly after bright flashes of light or have difficulty adjusting as light fades. In some parts of the world, such as Indonesia, where vitamin A deficiency is common, this condition is called "chicken eyes." This is because chickens can't see well at night and go to sleep when the sun sets.

Cellular Function

Vitamin A also plays another function of helping cells to mature and develop certain characteristics. This is ultimately crucial for a fetus to develop properly. In simple terms, vitamin A serves as a sort of traffic cop for cells, guiding them in their dividing and forming into the various tissues and organs that make up the body.

Immune Function

It is important to note that vitamin A is critical for proper immune function. It helps maintain the surfaces of the skin, mucous membranes lining the nose and throat, and the tissue linings of the intestines, bladder and other internal cavities. All of these benefits can help improve the immune response of the body because mucous membranes help prevent invasion by pathogens such as bacteria and viruses.

Vitamin A also helps play a more direct role in boosting immunity by aiding the various defense cells to change into the special forms required to fight off infections. For instance, the special T-helper cells, which help direct all other immunity cells, are extremely sensitive to vitamin A status. There is little question that the various immune cells and organs don't function very well when there is too little vitamin A. Some experts argue that you don't have to be clearly deficient for this occur.

Vitamin A is also involved in the health of bones, as it assists with the crucial process of bone regeneration. This process helps bones maintain their flexibility and strength.

Beta's Benefits

Given the wide-ranging responsibilities that vitamin A carries in the body, it's fortunate that we can get it from so many sources—plant as well as animal. While the transformation from beta carotene to vitamin A is complex, it doesn't take very long to occur.

In any case, the presence of beta carotene leads to the production of vitamin A as it is needed. And apart from its

CAROTENE CAUTION

Recent findings from different studies suggest that beta carotene may actually increase the risk of cancer among certain high-risk groups, most notably heavy smokers. This presents a special problem to scientists and doctors, because it raises questions about the exact functions of beta carotene and vitamin A, and why certain people may be at risk when taking supplements. It is important to note that many of these studies' participants were taking large doses of vitamin A, which we know can be toxic in excessive amounts. And of course, for each of these studies indicating possible detriment to taking beta carotene, there are dozens of other studies showing its wide-reaching health benefits.

So, what should you believe? Well, if you don't smoke, you probably shouldn't worry—there are plenty of reasons you should be taking beta carotene supplements. If you are a smoker, then quitting smoking would be the first and best course of action, followed by a commitment to a healthy diet, exercise and overall lifestyle plan. Of course, consulting with a health care practitioner qualified in these topics would also be a wise course of action. The bottom line is that while carotenes may pose a risk for a very small percentage of the population, they are known to have valuble benefits for the rest of us.

conversion to vitamin A, there is a large body of research indicating that beta carotene and the other carotenoids provide the body with a variety of other benefits, especially in the area of immunity and cancer prevention.

For years, researchers have noted that the more foods we eat that include carotenoids, especially beta carotene, the less likely we are to develop certain types of cancer, especially cancer of the lung, stomach, and esophagus. And recent studies have linked beta carotene to reduced risk of cervical and colon cancer as well.

Cancer Prevention

So how does beta carotene help prevent cancer? There may be several reasons, but two stand out. Researchers have determined that beta carotene possesses antioxidant properties. Like vitamins C and E and other antioxidants, beta carotene can neutralize the free-roaming unstable free radicals that cause cellular damage, which may ultimately lead to conditions like cancer.

It is also thought that beta carotene helps prevent cancer through its regulation of cell-to-cell communication. Every cell has the ability to communicate with its neighbors, just as if it were calling out across the backyard fence. When normal cells are grown within a laboratory, they won't pile up on top of one another once they have reached the top layer of a cell culture system. When the top layer is reached, the cells send messages to each other that in effect say, "We are done growing." Thus, all the cells in that culture stop dividing and growing.

BETA CAROTENE/VITAMIN A FAST FACTS

Possible Benefits: These two supplements fight cancer, suppressed immune function, colds, flu, heart disease, angina, vision problems, conditions related to oxidative damage, proper bone/teeth development, proper fetal development, allergies, and asthma.

Special Instructions: To avoid ingesting toxic amounts of vitamin A, stick with a mix of supplements that offer both vitamin A and beta carotene. Taking more beta carotene than vitamin A is usually the safer route. For optimal absorption, take supplements with food that contains some fat. Do not take with meals that contain high amounts of pectin, a type of fiber found mainly in citrus fruits. This can decrease the absorption of beta carotene supplements.

Dietary Sources: Beta carotene—orange and yellow fruits and vegetables, such as carrots, melons, squash and dark green, leafy vegetables such as spinach; Vitamin A—dairy products, eggs and meat products such as liver.

Who's at Risk for Deficiency?: Cigarette smokers, alcoholics, and those eating a poor diet (less than three servings of vegetables/fruits daily).

> *Cautions and Possible Side Effects:* Do not take preformed vitamin A supplements unless you are under supervision by a qualified health practitioner. Taking large amounts of preformed vitamin A for extended periods can lead to various health problems. If you are pregnant or nursing a child, do not take more than 8,000 IU of active vitamin A as this can be toxic to the child or cause birth defects. Taking beta carotene is quite safe, as most of any extra not used by the body is usually stored for later use. The only possible drawback of too much beta carotene (and it's not a dangerous thing) is a condition where the skin gains a tint of orange/yellow. If you wish to take therapeutic amounts of vitamin A for existing health conditions, see your doctor for supervision.

This is a fascinating phenomenon to cancer researchers because the exact opposite of this happens when cancer begins—the cells don't stop growing. Due to an apparent lack of communication, they just continue to grow and grow. In their frenetic growing process, they just "pile up," eventually forming tumors. As the growth continues, the cancerous cells invade the space of healthy cells and, in a sense, take over the neighborhood.

Though more research is needed, some findings indicate that beta carotene can in fact lower the risk of certain cancers, and researchers think this is at least partly due to its role in cell-to-cell communications.

Heart Disease

Several studies have shown that supplementing with beta carotene and vitamin A can have a significant impact on reducing the risk of heart-related conditions. One ongoing study has revealed that men with a history of heart disease who took beta carotene supplements cut in half the occurrence of heart attacks, strokes and deaths related to their conditions, as opposed to the other male patients not taking the supplements.

The Bottom Line

Most people know that both vitamin A and its precursor beta carotene are needed by the body. However, a growing body of research is making it more apparent that beta carotene especially can provide many vital and wide-ranging benefits, from cancer prevention to relief from colds/flu to fighting free radical damage. Couple this with the fact that it is more and more difficult to consume a healthy diet, and all of this adds up to making beta carotene one of today's top nutritional supplements for disease prevention and overall excellent health.

10

Fiber

HOPEFULLY EVERYONE KNOWS THAT fiber is an important part of a balanced diet. Fiber helps regulate the digestive system and contributes to a healthy colon. It helps prevent constipation, irritable bowel syndrome, diverticulitis and hemorrhoids. Along with those benefits, fiber may also help prevent colon and breast cancer, and decrease the risk of high cholesterol, diabetes and heart disease.

How It Works

Fiber is the indigestible part of all plant foods—fruits, vegetables, grains and beans. It is not found in meat or other animal foods. Fiber is roughage that cannot be digested. Depending on the type of food you eat, you may get either soluble or insoluble fiber. Soluble fiber dissolves in water and forms a gel-like substance in the stomach and intestinal tract. Insoluble fiber, on the other hand, does not dissolve, but it does hold onto water and moves quickly through the intestines. Many sources of fiber include both soluble and insoluble types. For example, the fiber in an apple is about 31 percent insoluble and 14 soluble. Both

---

FIBER FAST FACTS

Possible Uses: Helps prevent constipation, irritable bowel syndrome, diverticulitis, hemorrhoids, colon and breast cancer, high cholesterol, diabetes and heart disease.

Dietary Sources: Fruits, vegetables, whole grains, beans, seeds and nuts.

Dosages: 25 grams of fiber is the FDA daily recommended value (DRV). The American Dietetic Association (ADA) recommends between 20 and 35 grams per day. Some physicians recommend 40 grams to maintain optimal health.

Special Instructions: Be sure to drink plenty of water as you increase your fiber intake, as blockages can occur. Another result of large amounts of fiber is flatulence, and sometimes bloating. Introduce fiber slowly and experiment with different types and different amounts to find what is right for you. Be careful not to overdo it. Too much fiber can also decrease the absorption of certain nutrients.

types of fiber add bulk to the stool and get it out of the body sooner. Eliminating waste and toxins from the colon contributes greatly to overall health.

Fanatics for Fiber

If you need to be convinced of the value of fiber, listen to some of the ways that fiber benefits us. First, fiber absorbs sugars and starches from the small intestine, thus contributing to blood sugar regulation. This may help to ward off the onset of type 2 diabetes. Soluble fiber also binds to bile, of which cholesterol is an important ingredient. Fiber can lower blood cholesterol levels by at least 5 percent in people with healthy levels, and even more in those who have high cholesterol levels.

Insoluble fiber provides bulk that moves residue through the intestine. This helps prevent constipation and diverticular disease. Insoluble fiber also flushes carcinogens, bile acids and cholesterol from the body. Studies of total fiber intake (both soluble and insoluble) show a decreased risk of colon, rectal, breast, prostate and other cancers when the patients consume a high-fiber diet.

A final important reason to eat fiber is its role in weight management. Fiber helps you to feel full and slows the emptying of the stomach. High-fiber diets also tend to have fewer calories and contribute less to obesity. Lowering your weight can also lower your risk for the development of cancer, high blood pressure and diabetes.

Types of Fiber Supplements

Glucomannan

Glucomannan is one type of soluble fiber. It is derived from the konjac root (Amorphophallus konjac) and is considered a bulk-forming laxative. Glucomannan helps produce a larger, bulkier stool that passes through the colon more easily and requires less pressure to expel. Good results have been noted in studies using glucomannan to fight constipation. It helps produce a bowel movement within 12 to 24 hours in constipated individuals.

As with other fibers, glucomannan delays the emptying of the stomach, which leads to a more gradual absorption of dietary sugar. Studies involving people with diabetes show that overall control of sugar levels is improved when glucomannan is included in the daily diet. Glucomannan can also help lower cholesterol levels and fight obesity.

Psyllium

Another common type of soluble fiber is psyllium. Psyllium is a seed grown in India that is a common ingredient in laxatives. The seed is surrounded by a substance called mucilage that becomes gel-like once it reaches the digestive tract. Psyllium improves stool consistency, so it helps alleviate both constipation and diarrhea. Studies have shown that it even helps with the diarrhea caused by medications used to treat HIV.

Like other fibers, psyllium also helps lower blood cholesterol levels. Its high levels of soluble fiber may reduce the absorption of cholesterol. It is also important to note that the U.S. Food and Drug Administration (FDA) has approved psyllium to reduce cardiovascular disease after reviewing the results of recent studies. Similar to glucomannan, psyllium is also helpful for people with irritable bowel syndrome and colon inflammation. It also the subject of current studies that are investigating the benefits of psyllium for those with diabetes. One small study of 18 people showed good results, but more research is needed.

Modified Citrus Pectin

Modified citrus pectin is another form of fiber that is found principally in citrus fruits such as oranges and tangerines. It has been changed from its original form, which gives it potential action not found in normal pectin. Promising research has recently emerged showing that modified citrus pectin can stop the spread of prostate cancer and melanoma, though more research is probably needed to determine exactly how it works.

Oat Bran

During the 1980s, oat bran enjoyed a high level of publicity. Technically, oat bran is made by grinding the inner husk of the whole oat grain. Study after study confirmed that consistently eating oat bran can lower high blood serum cholesterol as much as 20 percent or more. Even already low blood cholesterol was shown to be reduced by 5 percent by consuming daily doses of oat bran.

> **FABULOUS FIBER**
>
> Dietary fiber has the ability to:
>
> - Increase fecal bulk by retaining water
> - Decrease stool transit time
> - Keep blood sugar levels more stable
> - Prevent weight gain by slowing the rate of digestion and absorption and by controlling hunger
> - Lower blood serum and liver cholesterol levels
> - Expedite the removal of potentially dangerous toxins and carcinogens from the bowel by acting as a carrier and by boosting elimination
> - Increase the production and presence of healthier intestinal bacteria

Of course, it must be understood that oat bran (and any other fiber) must be eaten consistently and indefinitely to maintain its ability to lower cholesterol. In addition, having a bowl of hot oat cereal and then eating a diet that is high in animal fats is not recommended. Remember that oatmeal, which is the ground version of the whole oat grain, contains about one third less fiber than the bran. Also, be careful not confuse the term "oat fiber" for "oat bran." Oat fiber additions to certain commercial products may originate from oat hulls, which is a type of insoluble fiber.

Give Your Heart a Hand

Fiber does much more than just contribute to a healthy colon. Various studies have shown that people who eat more fiber have less risk of heart disease. In a study that used 44,000 male health professionals as subjects, it was found that those who had more than 25 grams of fiber per day in their diet had a 36 percent lower risk of developing heart disease than those who ate 15 grams daily. Soluble fiber binds with bile acids and cholesterol in the intestinal tract, preventing their reabsorption. It is this process that helps lower blood cholesterol levels.

Keep It Regular

The best way to obtain fiber is to increase your intake of fruits, vegetables, whole grains, beans, seeds and nuts. Raspberries have a huge amount of fiber because of all the tiny seeds they contain. One cup of the fruit contains 40 grams of fiber. Half a cup of cooked beans has 4 grams of fiber—a nice contribution to your daily dosage of fiber. If you are constipated, try a fiber supplement, fluid and exercise as the answer to your problem.

Do You Need Fiber Supplements?

Actually getting enough fiber is problematic for many Americans. We often only eat about 14 or 15 grams of fiber, but 20 grams is the minimum we should be eating.

In fact, the deficiency of fiber in an ordinary diet is a significant health problem in our society. We know that five servings of fruits and vegetables is the minimum number a healthy adult should have in a normal day—yet how many servings did you have yesterday? The best way to obtain fiber is to increase your intake of fruits, vegetables, whole grains, beans, seeds and nuts. There are also pills, capsules and powders available. Be aware, however, that these may interfere with the absorption of minerals from foods. Taking straight wheat bran is also not advisable.

The Bottom Line

Forty or fifty years ago, the notion that refined grain flours, meat and dairy made up the ideal diet. We now know that diets high in whole foods—that is vegetables, fruits, whole grains, nuts and the like—are much more healthy, with their fiber content being a big part of that. Fiber is a marvelous multifaceted health agent. It can decrease your risk of certain cancers, heart disease, diabetes, and high blood pressure. It can fight and even reverse digestive ailments. It aids the body in proper utilization of nutrients, and maintains a healthy transit time. In short, fiber is vital for super health.

11

Green Tea

ONLY RECENTLY HAS the Western world discovered the benefits of drinking green tea that Asians have enjoyed for centuries. Green tea has its origins in China, and other Asian cultures have also adopted green tea as a common drink. For at least one thousand years these cultures have reaped many health benefits from drinking tea that is easily prepared and readily available.

Green tea has been highly valued for its medicinal uses from early times. We now know that the major chemical component of the tea leaf is a group of phytochemicals known as polyphenols. It is polyphenols that provide the health benefits for which green tea is used. Long known as tea tannin, polyphenols are extremely pungent and constitute 15 to 30 percent of dried green tea leaves. Green tea is processed in a way that protects polyphenols by destroying the enzyme that oxidizes them. But what does this mean for you? How can drinking green tea help you? You may be surprised at how much green tea can do for your body.

Asia's Hidden Healer

Green tea may be one of the most valuable substances you can take to protect your general health. The wide-reaching health benefits of green tea, all of which have been demonstrated in scientific studies, include:

- acting as a strong antioxidant.
- protecting against cancer.
- lowering cholesterol and blood pressure.
- working as an antibacterial and antiviral agent.

In fresh tea leaves, polyphenols exist as a series of chemicals called catechins, which include gallocatechin o(GC), epigallocatechin (EGC), epicatechin (EC), epigallocatechin gallate (EGCg), and epicatechin gallate (Ecg). These catechins function in ways to rid the body of toxins, lower levels of cholesterol, slow or stop blood pressure increase, and act as antibiotics.

Antioxidant Properties

Though oxygen is necessary for human life, it can be a harmful agent in the form of active oxygen, also known as free-radical oxygen. Active oxygen is a problem because it can combine with anything in the body and oxidize it, with consequent destruction of cell membranes, damage to DNA and oxidation of lipids (fats). All of these can lead

---

GREEN TEA FAST FACTS

Possible Benefits: Acts as an antioxidant, helps to protect against cancer, lowers cholesterol levels, stimulates the immune system, fights tooth decay, and may delay the onset of atherosclerosis.

Special Instructions: To get green tea's full benefits, drink it without milk, which may bind with some of the beneficial compounds and make them unavailable to the body. Although some experts suggest drinking 4-10 cups a day, if this seems like too much, supplement forms are available. Also, be aware that green tea does contain caffeine.

Forms available: Capsule, dried leaves, extract, and infusion (made from loose tea or tea bags).

Other Information: Because green tea is simply the dried leaves of the tea plant, it is much more effective as an antioxidant than black tea. Black tea undergoes natural fermentation, which converts the tannins into more complex compounds which destroys the polyphenols. Thus, black tea does not have the health benefits that green tea does.

to diseases like cancer or heart disease. As a result, it is necessary for us to provide our bodies with something that can counter this activity—some form of antitoxin or antioxidant.

The antioxidant component of green tea has been shown to efficiently scavenge free radical toxins. Green tea's antioxidant activity is particularly important for preventing lipid peroxidation, which often plays a key role in the buildup of arterial plaque. And green tea polyphenols have shown in studies to have greater antioxidant protection than powerhouse vitamins C and E. In addition to exerting antioxidant activity on its own, green tea increases the activity of the body's own antioxidant system, including activation of compounds like superoxide dismutase (SOD) and glutathione peroxidase.

Cancer Prevention

The anticancer effects of green tea are the result of polyphenols blocking the formation of cancer-causing compounds. In addition, these phytochemicals effectively detoxify or trap cancer-causing chemicals. In other words, they have the ability to halt enzymes that produce carcinogens and the ability to inhibit cancer growth.

The forms of cancer which appear to be prevented best by green tea are cancers of the gastrointestinal tract, including cancers of the stomach, small intestine, pancreas, and colon; lung cancer; and estrogen-related cancers, including breast cancer. In Japan, the popular custom of drinking green tea with meals is thought to be a major factor in the low rates of these types of cancer.

Although it is not clear exactly how green tea works to fight cancer, EGCg (the catechin of which green tea has the greatest amount) leads to the programmed cell death, or apoptosis, of cancer cells. It seems to communicate, through an as yet unknown cell-signaling pathway, to the cancer cells that they had better self-destruct or they will be destroyed. The cells make a decision and undergo apoptosis. This apoptosis shows up as a clear and distinct shape of the cells and in the breakdown of the molecular structure. Clearly, green tea can help to protect against cancer.

Cholesterol Control

Cholesterol is usually cited as a "bad guy" for causing various diseases in adults, but it is a chemical present in all animals and it is necessary for important body processes such as manufacturing cell membranes and fusing cells. There are two types of cholesterol: one is the cholesterol often referred to as "bad" (the LDL and VLDL type) and the other is labeled "good" cholesterol (the HDL type). LDL cholesterol accumulates in body tissue, while HDL cholesterol actually collects excessive cholesterol from the tissues.

If the amount of bad cholesterol in the blood becomes too much, it collects on blood vessel walls and can lead to atherosclerosis. Atherosclerosis, in conjunction with high blood pressure, cause heart disease. Good cholesterol can

> ### ANTIBACTERIAL AND ANTIVIRAL FIGHTER
>
> Tea catechins are strong antibacterial and antiviral agents which make them effective for treating everything from tooth decay to HIV. EGCg and other polyphenols in green tea have been shown to inhibit the spread of several types of bacteria in the respiratory tract. They have also been shown to effectively prevent the influenza virus from adhesion to normal cells, thus blocking flu infection. Even a small amount of EGCg seems to be able to significantly obstruct the flu virus. Finally, polyphenols act against infections caused by enterovirus, a common cause of diarrhea. Oral bacteria which causes tooth decay is also destroyed by green tea catechins. So green tea is good for oral hygiene.

help prevent atherosclerosis and should exist in proper balance for good health. The compounds in green tea have been shown to reduce levels of "bad" cholesterol in the blood—LDL-and VLDL cholesterol—and to increase the "good" HDL cholesterol. Green tea catechin also restricts excessive buildup of blood cholesterol.

Blood Pressure Reduction

High blood pressure is known to give the vascular system serious problems and contribute to atherosclerosis.

Atherosclerosis can then initiate heart disease, stroke, and other cardiovascular diseases. The cause of high blood pressure is not yet fully understood, but it is known that a compound angiotensin II plays a role in high blood pressure.

In hypertension caused by high blood pressure, angiotensin I converting enzyme (ACE) converts angiotensin I to vasoconstrictive angiotensin II. When this process is blocked, it is possible to prevent hypertension to a large extent. This is the mechanism that ACE-inhibitor drugs use to treat high blood pressure. There are, however, other effective means to treat high blood pressure. Studies have shown green tea polyphenols to have significant ACE-inhibiting ability. They reduce blood pressure to make heart disease and stroke less likely.

The Bottom Line

The health benefits of green tea are varied and wide-ranging. Because the chemical makeup of green tea gives it the capability to positively affect so many different systems in the body, it makes sense to use it in achieving a better state of health. What Asians have known for centuries about drinking green tea can now benefit the world.

12

Coenzyme Q10

SAD BUT TRUE—as we age, our bodies begin to lose the ability to manufacture many of the substances required for optimal health. Coenzyme Q10 (also known as co Q10) is one of those substances. Coenzyme Q10 is made by the body and stored in the liver, kidneys, pancreas and heart. It is found in all cells, but the cells of the heart contain the most because they use the greatest amount of energy.

What Exactly Is Co Q10?

There are actually ten substances known as coenzyme Qs, but coenzyme Q10 is the only one found in human tissue. It is similar to a vitamin, and is critical in the production of energy at the cellular level. Coenzyme Q10 also stimulates the immune system, has vital anti-aging effects, and helps with circulation.

How Does It Work?

Every cell in the body contains mitochondria, and mitochondria contains genetic material and many enzymes that are important for cell metabolism. This includes those responsible for the conversion of food to usable energy. One of the most important is coenzyme Q10. What it does is contribute to the production of ATP, which is the immediate source of energy for cells. ATP increases energy and stamina, builds muscles, fights fatigue, and preserves muscle fibers. Coenzyme Q10 carries protons and electrons into each cell and they are used to create ATP. This process is never ending because the body can only store a small amount of ATP.

The Need for Supplementation

It has been shown that as many as 75 percent of people over the age of fifty may be deficient in coenzyme Q10. This is a frightening statistic because a lack of this substance can contribute to heart disease. Without coenzyme Q10 the heart does not have enough energy to circulate blood effectively. Most of us have sufficient coenzyme Q10 until we are about age thirty, and then levels begin to diminish.

The people who have the most severe lack of coenzyme Q10 are those with various types of heart disease. What doctors don't know is whether the lack of the enzyme contributes to heart disease or is the result of heart disease.

Regardless, coenzyme Q10 is definitely a factor in heart disease, and what numerous studies have shown is that as you supplement and restore levels of the enzyme to where they need to be, heart function improves. With appropriate levels of coenzyme Q10 there is enhanced energy production, the heart has better ability to contract, and antioxidant protection increases. The activity of coenzyme Q10 also helps prevent the buildup of LDL, or "bad," cholesterol.

Fighting Parkinson's Disease

Research has shown that people with Parkinson's disease have low levels of coenzyme Q10 and that the function of the mitochondria in their cells is impaired. In a 2002 study, ten hospitals across the United States were involved in a test using coenzyme Q10 to treat Parkinson's. Eighty patients who were in the early stages of the disease were placed randomly in one of four groups. Each group was given a different dosage of the compound—1200 mg, 600 mg, 300 mg, or a placebo. After eight months of taking coenzyme Q10 the differences in the groups first began to show. After sixteen months, the study determined that the people taking the highest dosage of coenzyme Q10 had 44 percent less decline in their ability to do daily activities, such as walking, bathing and dressing. Even though the study involved a relatively small number of patients, the results show great hope in the treatment of Parkinson's using a natural compound already found in the body.

The Added Bonus

Research has shown that supplementing with coenzyme Q10 not only helps the heart and fights aging, it also has the ability to counter histamine. Histamine is released in the body as part of an allergic reaction in humans. It causes dilation of capillaries (that's why we have red eyes), constriction of bronchial smooth muscle (makes it difficult to breathe), and decreased blood pressure (can cause

---

COENZYME Q10 FAST FACTS

Possible Benefits: Protects and strengthens the heart, helps treat high blood pressure and other cardiovascular diseases, strengthens muscles, stimulates the immune system, and fights against aging diseases.

Forms Available: Capsule, liquid, and oil. Gel capsules are readily absorbed and easy to swallow. Coenzyme Q10 is best absorbed when taken with fatty foods, such as fish or peanut butter. Recommendations vary from 60 to 120 mg twice daily.

Cautions and Possible Side Effects: Coenzyme Q10 has a safe history, and almost never has side effects. In rare cases, stomach upset, diarrhea, and nausea have been reported.

dizziness). People who suffer from allergies, asthma or other respiratory ailments can benefit from taking coenzyme Q10.

The Bottom Line

Younger people probably have all the coenzyme Q10 their body needs, so paying a good amount of money for supplements is probably not worth it for them. However, as we age, we can help maintain the youth of our heart by providing it with a substance that makes it stronger. It is interesting to note that more than twelve million Japanese take coenzyme Q10 at the direction of their physicians. As Americans learn more about the value of this important compound, the numbers of doctors and patients both using and supporting the use of coenzyme Q10 will only increase.

13

Soy Isoflavones

As is the case with other supplements, people often wonder if it is as effective to receive the benefits of soy through supplements as it is through soy food products. While the answer to this question can be debated, it is becoming increasingly clear that soy supplements containing one or more isoflavones—particularly genistein—can provide many if not all of the same benefits that come from eating foods derived from soy.

Over the last few years, soy foods such as tofu, milk, flour, miso, tempeh and protein have become largely mainstream products. Many soy-derived foods can be found at your local grocery store, pharmacy and health food store. During this same time, piles of research have confirmed that soy can help the body in many ways, from strengthening bones to relieving menopausal discomforts to fighting cancer.

Now there are emerging products containing soy extracts, principally what are called *isoflavones*, which exert estrogen-like effects in the body, albeit in a more mild manner. Because they are structurally similar to estrogen, isoflavones can produce the benefits of estrogen yet avoid some of the dangerous aspects of estrogen, such as increased cancer risk.

Minimizing Menopause Discomfort

For many women, the prospect of going through menopause is a confusing and frightening one. Myths and misinformation abound, especially regarding the best ways to fight the discomforts that come with menopause. Now in light of the recent reports from government agencies showing that the risks of using synthetic hormone replacement therapy (HRT) drugs outweigh the benefits, women are left even more in the dark about how to proceed.

There is an impressive body of research demonstrating that soy and its main components can provide relief from common menopausal discomforts. A number of studies have demonstrated that soy can significantly reduce the number and severity of hot flashes, while others have shown that soy isoflavones can reduce the rates of night sweats as well. Additionally, the research teams for many of these studies have recommended that soy and its compounds be considered for use in treating menopausal symptoms, especially for women suffering from mild to moderate symptoms.

Genistein and Cancer Prevention

The prospect of developing cancer related to hormonal activity, like breast and ovarian cancer, is a major fear among middle-age and older women. Genistein and other soy isoflavones have shown impressive results in fighting cancer. Research shows that it does this in a variety of ways:

- First, genistein has only about one-thousandth the hormone potency of estrogen. So it helps prevent cancer when it attaches to the estrogen receptor sites of breast cells, which prevents the much more potent and potentially dangerous estrogen from attaching to these same receptor sites.

- Another way that genistein works to prevent cancer is through slowing down activity of the hypothalamus and pituitary gland, which both contribute to the production of estrogen by the ovaries. So, the less estrogen flowing through the body, the longer a woman's cycle lasts, which translates to fewer cycles over her lifetime. Ultimately this means that her exposure to estrogen will be less, thereby decreasing her risk of breast cancer and other conditions.

- Research shows that genistein and other soy isoflavones are powerful antioxidants, which are considered to be a prime defense against cancer. Studies have also demonstrated that genistein may increase the production of superoxide dismutase (SOD), a potent antioxidant, and that may actually mimic the behavior of SOD in the body.

- Genistein contributes to apoptosis, or programmed cell death, which regulates all cell growth by not allowing them to reproduce too quickly. Researchers believe that genistein helps control tumor growth by enhancing this mechanism.

- Studies have also shown that genistein and other isoflavones can inhibit angiogenesis, the process by which new blood vessels are formed to feed tumors. If this process is stopped, the tumors actually become nutrient-starved and shrink.

- There is also some indication that genistein may help the mammary gland cells to mature and diversify, thereby cutting the risk of cancer. The mammary glands of women who have never nursed are more immature and thereby more vulnerable to cancer formation.

Soy and PMS Relief

Many women suffering from the monthly effects of premenstrual syndrome (PMS) have seen tremendous benefits from incorporating soy and soy supplements into their diet. PMS manifests itself to varying degrees through a variety of symptoms, including acne, bloating, backache, fatigue, extreme irritability, headache, sore or enlarged breasts, and depression, among others. Several studies have shown that soy foods and supplements can have a beneficial impact on the effects of PMS. In short, the increased presence of isoflavones occupying the estrogen receptor sites causes a decrease in circulating estrogen. Lower levels of estrogen are known to result in fewer or less severe symptoms of PMS.

SOY ISOFLAVONE FAST FACTS

Possible Benefits: Reducing risk of breast and ovarian cancer, relief from effects of PMS, relief of menopausal symptoms, including hot flashes and night sweats, reducing risk of cardiovascular disease, reversing/preventing osteoporosis

Product Forms: Tablets are capsules are probably the most common forms. They are usually marketed under the names "soy isoflavones," "isoflavones," or "genistein." Look for products that offer a guaranteed, standardized level of isoflavone content, especially genistein and daidzein.

Dietary Sources: Various soy-derived foods, including tofu, miso, tempeh, soy milk, soy flour, soy proteins, and whole soy beans

Heart Health: It's in the Isoflavones

Numerous studies have shown that soy, and in particular its isoflavones, can benefit the heart and cardiovascular system in several different ways. And so impressive are its heart-healthy attributes that in 2000, the FDA allowed soy food products to carry a health claim stating that soy is effective in fighting coronary heart disease. While results have been mixed, there is promising research surrounding both genistein and daidzein and their complementary effect in fighting heart disease.

Building Better Bones

Researchers around the world are very excited about soy's ability to strengthen bones, increase bone mass and prevent osteoporosis. One reason is that soy is a great dietary source of calcium. As you probably know, calcium is essential for healthy bones and proper development of the musculoskeletal system. Another reason is that genistein and daidzein appear to inhibit the breakdown of bones. One study showed that soy isoflavones helped fortify bones found in the lumbar spine and also prevented the development of dowager's hump, which is commonly seen in postmenopausal women. Another study demonstrated that genistein aided in the retention of bone mineral mass equivalent to prescription doses of estradiol.

> **SOY IN THE HEADLINES**
>
> "Soy Cuts Insulin, Cholesterol in Diabetic Women"
> *ABC News*
>
> "Diet Rich in Soy Protein Lowers Estrogens Associated with Breast Cancer"
> *Intelihealth*
>
> "Soy Isoflavone May Improve Bone Metabolism"
> *Doctor's Guide*
>
> "Soy Isoflavone May Be Safe, Effective Alternative to Estrogen Replacement"
> *Medscape*
>
> "FDA Approves Soy Health Claims for Heart Disease"
> *Women's Health*
>
> "Soy May Decrease Cancer Risks"
> *Science Daily*

Soy's Other Health Benefits

Aside from the benefits surrounding hormone-related conditions in women, heart disease and cancer, soy and its principal components are showing promise in helping other areas, including the following:

- Fighting bacterial and fungal infections
- Acting as a diuretic
- Improving kidney function
- Relieving effects of type II diabetes
- Preventing gallstones

The Bottom Line

Soy not only offers hormonal health to women young and old, it also provides powerful antioxidant protection against cancer, as well as promoting heart health. In fact, the benefits of soy are so wide-reaching, that nearly everyone would benefit from supplementation, whether they are currently healthy or suffering from chronic disease.

14

Garlic

AFTER STUDYING TO BECOME a doctor, Albert Schweitzer decided he wanted to dedicate his life to helping improve the life of others. In order to pursue his goal, he traveled to Africa and lived the remainder of his life there, eventually winning the Nobel Prize in recognition of his efforts. Interestingly, one of the remedies that Dr. Schweitzer often used during his time in Africa was garlic. He knew of the antibiotic qualities of garlic, and applied them in his treatment of amebic dysentery. Later, during World War II, garlic was often used when supplies of penicillin ran short. Soldiers would use the juice of garlic as treatment for infected wounds.

But Dr. Pasteur and WWII soldiers were hardly the first people to recognize the value of garlic. Garlic has been used for thousands of years by various cultures—from the Egyptian pharaohs to the Chinese emperors. Today, in

Korea, garlic is eaten at almost every meal, and the Koreans are quick to point out the myriad benefits of garlic.

What Makes Garlic Great?

Garlic is a member of the Allium family. Other members of this family are onions, leeks, shallots, and chives. The most potent compound in garlic is called allicin. Chemists first isolated allicin about sixty years ago, and since then interest in its medicinal properties has not waned. Allicin is a pungent and strongly antibiotic compound and most people pay attention to allicin as the indicator of garlic's value.

The Many Roles of Garlic

Garlic is used for a wide variety of ailments. Long ago, European peasants wore it around their necks to ward off vampires and other evil spirits. Because vampires do not usually bother people today, garlic is used for other problems such as colds, coughs, flu, chronic bronchitis, dysentery, asthma, intestinal worms, dysentery, and fever.

Since the 1960s, hundreds of scientific studies have been done that investigate garlic and other plants from the same family. Garlic has been found to affect blood pressure and cholesterol levels, and it helps to thin the blood. These three qualities make garlic a wise supplement choice for people who are at risk for heart attack. But that is not all. Garlic fights against bacteria in the stomach, and some scientists believe that it can work to prevent gastric cancer. Besides its anti-cancer properties, garlic also works as an anti-inflammatory, and has antibiotic, antiviral, antifungal and antiseptic properties.

Give a Stinking Rose to Your Heart

Garlic, called "the stinking rose" by the Greeks and the Romans, has a five-thousand-year history of culinary and medicinal use. Aside from its employment in the kitchen, garlic is most often used to treat conditions that affect the heart. When plaque (a fatty deposit) builds up in the arteries, the blood flow to the heart and brain can be reduced. Clots can form, or bits of plaque may form blockages. When this happens, a heart attack or stroke can result. Garlic benefits the heart and the circulatory system in a number of ways.

Dutch researchers conducted over twenty studies showing that five or more cloves of fresh garlic a day lowers cholesterol levels, thus reducing the risk of heart disease. Luckily, you don't have to eat that much fresh garlic to enjoy its effects. Taking a pill or a powder of the equivalent amount will do the trick. One study found that after only four weeks of taking garlic tablets, participants had a 5 to 6 percent reduction in total cholesterol levels. In another study, twenty healthy people took garlic oil twice a day for six months. Their blood cholesterol levels fell significantly.

Garlic and the Stomach

Along with helping your heart, garlic can also contribute to the happiness of your stomach. It has been discovered that a common bacteria called *H. pylori* appears to be involved in the development of stomach

---

GARLIC FAST FACTS

Possible Benefits: Relief of stomach and intestinal upset, colds, coughs, flu, bronchitis, fevers, ringworm, and asthma. Also used to treat atherosclerosis, high blood pressure, high cholesterol and blood clots.

Forms: Fresh garlic is easily obtained. However, if you feel your social life may suffer from its aroma, there are other forms available: capsule, extract, infusion, liquid, tablet, oil and juice. There is also a supplement called aged garlic extract (AGE). It has been shown in some studies that the aging process substantially boosts garlic's antioxidant properties.

Cautions and Possible Side Effects: Do not take garlic if you have diabetes, as it may interfere with blood-sugar-lowering medications. Women who are pregnant or nursing should not take large amounts of garlic. Eating a dish flavored with garlic is fine, but be careful taking extra doses.

cancer and peptic ulcers. In laboratory tests, researchers have been able to kill *H. pylori* with garlic extract. Supplementing with garlic can help maintain the health of the intestinal tract. Garlic is dangerous for many types of bacteria, not just *H. pylori*, and has been found to affect bacteria that does not even respond to standard antibiotics.

Garlic—The Unadvertised Antioxidant

Another important, though often overlooked, fact about garlic is that it functions as an antioxidant. Science has long recognized the negative effects of free-radicals—unstable molecules in our bodies that lead to cell damage and aging. Free radicals may also contribute to the growth of tumors and cancer cells. Substances that counteract the effects of free radicals are called antioxidants. Common antioxidants are vitamins C and E, beta carotene, and selenium. Another supplement with powerful antioxidant properties is garlic. Studies involving laboratory animals have shown garlic to inhibit the growth of cancer cells. It has also been shown that the sulfur and hydrogen found in garlic bind with toxic heavy metals in the body so those metals can be excreted. Garlic also aids in detoxification and helps prevent dangerous fat deposits in tissues and arteries.

The Bottom Line

Garlic is an age-old remedy whose effects are supported by modern-day research. Use garlic for all its properties: antioxidant, anti-cancer, anti-inflammatory, antibiotic, antiviral, antifungal and antiseptic, and enjoy better health.

15

Olive Leaf Extract

WE'RE ALL NOW quite familiar with the problems stemming from the overuse of antibiotics—increased resistance by bacteria to many antibiotics, the development of more insidious "superbugs," the destruction by the antibiotic of beneficial bacteria, and the high risk of secondary infections. News headlines and magazine articles have been preaching the dangers of antibiotics for several years, and the public and medical world are both finally listening. We've recently seen the emergence of several "natural" antibiotics—botanicals and other compounds that not only fight bacteria, but viruses, fungi and other microbes as well.

One such natural medicine is olive leaf, whose extract has been used in various cultures for centuries to treat ailments from infected wounds to arthritis to heart disease. In fact, there is historical mention of olive leaf use as far back as the ancient Egyptians, who employed the leaf in their mummification rituals of their kings. Of course, early Mediterranean cultures used the olive leaf (and fruit) for nutritional and medicinal purposes.

Late in the 19th century, scientists began investigating olive leaf's medicinal properties and isolated a phenolic compound they ended up calling *oleuropein*. Most researchers considered this the component most responsible for olive leaf's therapeutic abilities. Then, in 1962 an Italian research team reported that oleuropein lowered blood pressure in animals, setting off a rush of investigative research targeting olive leaf and its potential as a medicinal agent.

The subsequent results from this research were certainly promising. European teams confirmed the finding that oleuropein could lower blood pressure, improve blood flow in prevent intestinal muscle spasms and relieve arrhythmia.

Old Remedy, New Uses

While olive leaf has been used for thousands of years in the Mediterranean and other cultures, it has only recently been a hot commodity in the U.S. And while long-term perspectives on its use are unclear, the results from initial studies are promising. More modern research on olive leaf extract has shown the following benefits:

- Another constituent of olive leaf, elenolic acid, has demonstrated impressive antiviral properties. Studies carried out by the pharmaceutical company Upjohn in the late 1960s indicated that elenolic acid was successful in inhibiting the growth of every virus it was tested against.

- Other recent research has shown that olive leaf is very effective at fighting bacterial infection, most likely by

---

OLIVE LEAF FAST FACTS

Possible Benefits: Improved immune function, protection against microbes, including bacteria, viruses, fungi, parasites, and yeast, protection against heart disease, high blood pressure, and improved energy, fibromyalgia, chronic fatigue syndrome, other autoimmune disorders

Product Forms: Capsules, tablets, tea

Special Instructions: The most current literature suggests that you should look for products with a guaranteed standard of 5–23 percent oleuropein per dose. Teas are not thought to be as effective as the guaranteed potency capsules or tablets.

Safety Issues: Olive leaf is very safe, especially when used in accordance with proper dosage guidelines. If you have concerns about using it, you should consult your doctor, especially if you are going to use it treat an existing condition.

dissolving the outer wall of individual bacterial cells.

- Another form of elenolic acid, called *calcium elenolate*, has generated interest because of its apparent ability to fight an array of bacteria, virus and fungal agents.

- Pharmacologists at the University of Granada discovered that olive leaf extract can promote the relaxation of the arterial walls. In addition to preventing heart disease, this finding also corroborates other research suggesting that olive leaf may be pivotal in fighting high blood pressure.

- Researchers at the University of Milan and elsewhere found that oleuropein inhibits oxidation of low-density lipoproteins, the "bad" cholesterol involved in the formation of various types of heart disease.

Natural Cold and Flu Relief

None of us likes to have the runny nose, cough, fever, aches and other symptoms that accompany the common cold and flu. And while usually these symptoms are more or less annoying, they can cost us valuable time at work and home. And for a few of us like the elderly and young children, the cold or flu can represent dangerous path to more serious conditions like pneumonia.

Aside from over-the-counter remedies that simply mask symptoms (and prolong suffering, according to several studies), there isn't much that conventional medicine has to offer. That's where "unconventional" therapies such as olive leaf can step in. Research shows that it can inhibit the action of a long list of viruses, bacteria, and other microbes, including (but not limited to) the following:

- *E.coli*
- *Bacillus cereus*
- *K. pneumoniae*
- *Candida albicans*
- Herpes
- Polio 1,2,3
- Retrovirus
- Moloney Murine leukemia
- Various influenza/parainfluenza viruses
- *Staphyloccus aureus*
- *Bacillus subtilis*
- *Cryptosporidium*
- *Giardia*
- Malaria-causing protozoa
- *Salmonella tyhimurium*
- *Pseudomonas fluorescens*

Working through various processes, olive leaf either inhibits viral/bacterial invaders, destroys them directly or stimulates the body's immune response to better handle the pathogens by itself. In these ways, olive leaf can provide protection from a variety of infections that plague us today.

Helpful for the Heart

Another area of high interest regarding olive leaf is that of protecting the heart and cardiovascular system. As mentioned earlier, research has shown that olive leaf extract may lower high blood pressure through dilating the coronary arteries. At least one study suggests that olive leaf can help constricted arteries relax and become more flexible, thereby for allowing for more blood flow (close to 50 percent more) and reducing blood pressure.

Other studies have produced other promising findings. One study focusing on oleuropein showed that it was effective in relieving barium chloride-induced arrhythmia, calcium-induced arrhythmia, as well as inducing a long-lasting effect of lowering elevated blood pressure.

Another way that olive leaf may benefit the heart and vascular system is through its antioxidant action. Various studies confirm that different constituents of olive leaf can effectively fight free radicals and prevent the oxidation of cholesterol in the arteries, and researchers attribute the lower levels of heart disease to this.

Energy, Blood Sugar and Olive Leaf

Besides helping fight microbes and prevent heart disease, olive leaf offers numerous other benefits as well. For instance, researchers in Spain found that olive leaf could have a significant effect on the management of blood sugar levels in hypoglycemics and diabetics. The researchers

> ## THE HERXHEIMER OR "DIE-OFF" EFFECT
>
> When people wonder if there are any side effects or safety concerns regarding olive leaf, the answer is generally a forceful "no." However, when olive leaf is being used to fight a chronic condition, there sometimes occur an adverse, albeit healthy, condition. This is generally referred to as the Herxheimer or "die-off" effect. What is this "die-off" effect? Simply put, it is the result of the toxic effect put off by the large number of pathogens (bacteria, virus, fungi, etc.) that are destroyed by olive leaf. Symptoms of this die-off include headache, muscle ache, swelling in the mouth, throat and lymphatics, rashes, fatigue, diarrhea, and other flu-like symptoms. Obviously, the severity of the effect will vary person to person, the state of their immune system and how much olive leaf they are consuming.
>
> However uncomfortable this may appear, it is actually desirable because it is a great indication that a beneficial change is occurring in the body. Needless to say, anyone who goes through this die-off usually feels fantastic afterwards, many times better than before.

believe that it can either stimulate the production of new insulin or increase the utilization of blood sugar in the body's extremities.

One of the most frequent comments reported by doctors from patients taking olive leaf is that they experience a dramatic increase in energy levels and have a greater sense of well-being. (In fact, some see such improved energy that they wonder if there is some sort of "upper" ingredient in olive leaf.) Improvement in energy levels has also been seen by many doctors in "fatigue" types of disorders, including chronic fatigue syndrome, fibromyalgia, lupus, Epstein-Barr, mononucleosis, and the like.

There are a number of health conditions for which olive leaf has shown promise. They include arthritis, AIDS, herpes, and other autoimmune disorders.

The Bottom Line

In today's world of poor diets, the evolution of "superbugs," high stress levels, toxic environments, an emphasis on antibiotics and other pharmaceutical drugs and overall poor lifestyles, natural agents like olive leaf can be a lifesaver. This herb can have a wide-reaching effect, protecting the body against invaders, preventing and lessening the effects of common ailments, fighting heart disease and hypertension, and improving energy levels. So look for some olive leaf today and make it part of your home medicine chest.

16

Saw Palmetto

IF YOU'VE HEARD anything about saw palmetto, you probably know it's mainly a "guy" herb. And the guys most likely to want it are middle-age or older men who find themselves needing to urinate more than they should, especially at night.

Typically, this call of nature usually ends up being a false alarm. Even when it feels like the bladder is about to burst, what typically occurs is a small trickle. This is a classic symptom of BPH, or benign prostatic hyperplasia, which is a noncancerous enlargement of the prostate gland. The enlargement of the prostate presses on and constricts the urethra, the tube that leads from the bladder to the penis, thereby making it difficult for urine to leave the bladder. Picture what happens to your garden sprinkler when you step on the garden hose, and you have a good idea of the problem.

All in all, a man's chance of developing BPH in his lifetime is very high, and his chances for prostate cancer are similarly high. Keeping in mind that a man's risk of developing prostate problems are very high, there are many steps he can take to prevent the development of these two diseases, and implementing a regimen of nutritional supplements, including saw palmetto, should be a big part of that.

Many men who take the herb discover that it lessens the inflammation of the prostate gland, thereby releasing the "squeeze" on the urethra so that the urine can flow normally and alleviating the often annoying and painful sensations that were previously common.

How well does it work? It's difficult to say exactly, but it is recognized as being at least helpful for moderate cases of BPH or a beginning case, and many experts tout it as being extremely helpful, even for more extreme cases.

Saw Palmetto: Its Common Uses

Saw palmetto is a scrubby palm that grows in the southeastern United States, from South Carolina to Florida. The Seminole Indians in Florida used the berries from the plant for food, and most likely, for some medicinal purposes. There are historical accounts of European settlers in the area using the plant as a diuretic and as an "anticatarrhal," meaning that it could relieve phlegm-producing conditions such as colds or respiratory infections. Women also employed it for painful periods and to regulate the menstrual cycle.

Saw palmetto can stimulate the production of prolactin, a female hormone that promotes the growth of breast tissue and milk production in lactating women. There are even reports of the herb showing benefit for infertility problems if the cause involves the absence of ovulation on the woman's part.

In the early part of this century, saw palmetto berries were widely used to treat urinary tract ailments, particularly chronic cystitis, an inflammation of the bladder. In fact, from 1906 to 1950, it was officially listed as a drug in the United States. After World War II, it began to fall out of favor in here, but research and widespread use continued in European countries. Researchers there discovered that patients consuming extracts of the berries had a beneficial increase in their urine volume, a decrease in their frequency of urination, and relief of burning, pressure and other discomforts during urination.

Saw Palmetto and BPH

As with some botanicals, it's difficult to know exactly how saw palmetto works, or what active ingredients are responsible for its benefits. Many scientists believe that saw palmetto demonstrates a steroidlike property. And in the case of BPH, it interrupts a critical chemical process. BPH occurs when the male hormone testosterone is converted by an enzyme to a more portent form of the hormone that causes cells to grow and proliferate. This growth is a perfectly normal thing when the male sexual organs are still growing and developing. But later in life, after development should have stopped, the continued cell growth in the prostate becomes a liability. If saw palmetto is taken regularly, it appears to inhibit the enzyme that encourages the hormone conversion.

SAW PALMETTO FAST FACTS

Possible Benefits: Benign prostatic hyperplasia (BPH), other prostate ailments, genitourinary ailments, impotence, painful periods

Product Availability: Saw palmetto is available in capsules, soft gel capsules, liquids and standardized extracts. Look for products that are standardized to an 85 to 95 percent fatty acid and sterol content. You may also find it teamed with other treatments like pygeum, zinc or pumpkin seeds in a combination product.

Safety Issues: Saw palmetto has been shown to be very safe, resulting in extremely few side effects, and producing no serious side effects, even with long-term use.

Special Instructions: It is vital that you consult with your physician concerning use of saw palmetto to verify that you indeed have BPH and not a more serious condition like cancer.

Several studies, especially several done in Europe, have shown that saw palmetto (primarily extracts of the berries) is an effective treatment for many men with BPH, especially those in the early stages of enlarged prostate. In one particular study, Belgian researchers found that saw palmetto benefited the prostate in various ways. Most notable was that it did not give misleadingly low prostate specific antigen (PSA) levels. Some pharmaceutical drugs given to treat BPH (Proscar in particular) can mask the markers indicating prostate cancer. The researchers state, "Our study clearly demonstrated the absence of such a risk with the administration of *Serenoa repens* [saw palmetto] extract, as the agent does not modify the serum PSA concentration." This study also found that the size of the prostate was significantly decreased—by about 10 percent—and that both patients and their physicians agreed that the herb was effective in relieving their symptoms. And just as important was that the herb resulted in discontinuation of treatment in only 2 percent of the subjects, a very low number compared to standard drug treatments. In an earlier study done by the same researchers, side effect levels were extremely low—fewer patients reported side effects than did the placebo group.

Many experts tout the very low level of side effects produced by saw palmetto as being its biggest selling point. While standard drugs may produce relatively better results with the BPH itself, they also produce significantly more side effects, so much so that a large percentage cannot take the drugs. Proscar, or its generic form finasteride, can cause headaches, erection problems, loss of sexual drive and decreased ejaculation volume. If you have tried these medications and have experienced undue side effects, then saw palmetto offers a safe, viable alternative.

Other Prostate Friends

Besides saw palmetto, there are a number of other natural agents that improve the health of the prostate and possibly relieve symptoms of BPH. Many experts recommend taking these in conjunction with saw palmetto to ensure that the prostate is receiving all the care it needs. These agents include the herb *Pygeum africanum* (typically called *pygeum*), zinc, pumpkin seeds, nettle, and fish oils/other essential fatty acids. It is also imperative that a healthy diet is followed and toxin intake, such as smoking, alcohol and unnecessary pharmaceutical drugs be minimized.

The Bottom Line

Although best known for its prostate protection, saw palmetto is actually a great supplement for both men and women. Keep this in your medicine cabinet if you or your family suffer from urinary tract infections, impotence, or painful periods. You might also try it for a boost in sex drive.

17

Calcium

CHALK, EGGSHELLS, AND MILK all have something in common—they get their dense white color from the same source—the mineral calcium. And they're loaded with it! Sharing this natural resource sometimes creates an interesting sort of lend-lease arrangement. Bones and eggshells are often ground and utilized in cattle feed; then, from milk and other dairy products that those cows provide, humans obtain some of the calcium they need for healthy bones, teeth and other tissues. If we don't get quite enough, we can turn to supplements.

There is more calcium than any other mineral in our bodies, and we're correct to associate it with bones, because that's where 99 percent of calcium is found. Adequate calcium levels are essential for building strong bones and teeth. But calcium is needed for more than this. It is also dissolved in the fluids in the body, bathing the cells inside and out. At the cellular level calcium helps muscles spring into action and aids the blood in clotting. It assists in the transmission of nerve impulses and launches hormones and enzymes on their journeys to organs and tissues throughout the body.

One important point to know about calcium is that although most Americans usually don't suffer from such low levels of calcium that these basic processes are impaired, our bodies sometimes are forced to act like poachers during lean times. If there is not enough calcium present, then our bodies simply rob calcium from bones to ensure that these vital functions continue.

Bones: Rock Hard . . . Or Not

Most of us are aware of the high risk of osteoporosis among older people, especially women. Osteoporosis is a condition marked by porous, brittle bones that break easily. Contrary to what many of us imagine, healthy bones aren't inert, rocklike objects. They are in a state of constant change, dissolving and forming new bone tissue all the time.

As bones begin to form, calcium salts form crystals on a gridwork of protein strands called collagen. These crystals form in and around the collagen, gradually lending more strength and rigidity to the developing tissue. The time that this happens most often and fastest is during childhood and adolescence, or when a broken bone is under repair. Bones reach their peak mass—when they're most

WHICH CALCIUM IS BEST?

If you are considering taking calcium supplements, you won't find a shortage of products. Be aware, however, that most multivitamin/mineral products don't have much calcium because it's so bulky and is hard to fit in with the rest of the ingredients. Calcium comes from a variety of natural sources, including bone, oyster shells, limestone, and more recently, coral. Manufacturers purify the calcium to varying degrees or combine them with other compounds, like gluconate or citrate.

Based on limited research, it appears that supplements of calcium combined with amino acids, or calcium gluconate, lactate or citrate are the best-absorbed forms. These are usually taken between meals, but you may need to experiment with this if you experience an upset stomach.

If you are considering calcium supplements for an existing condition, it would be wise to consult with a qualified practitioner familiar with calcium supplements, their various forms, and their interactions/functions within the body. This way, you can ensure that the calcium supplement you end up taking is the one you need most.

One other thing to remember that no matter what form of calcium you take, it is vital that you take additional magnesium and vitamin D. This will ensure that the calcium is properly absorbed and utilized.

dense and strongest—in your late twenties. Thus, it is crucial that we get enough calcium early on—the more dense your bones are at their peak, the longer they'll maintain their strength and density.

And it's just as important to maintain a steadily high intake of calcium well after your peak years. This will help offset the loss of bone mass that naturally occurs as you age.

Muscle and Nerve Function

Calcium is also vitally important for proper muscle and nerve functioning. In order to contract and then relax, the muscles depend on adequate levels of calcium to be present. If you have too little calcium present in your muscles, they tend to stay in a tightened (contracted) state. This can make you prone to cramps.

Along with other electrically aggressive minerals like potassium, calcium allows our nerves to transmit messages. Calcium ions in the cell move from one spot to another very quickly, changing the electrical charge or certain proteins in the muscle. This is necessary for muscle contraction/extension as well as nerve transmission. As the ions shift quickly, an electrical charge is handed along the chain of nerve cells. This results in a small electrical current traveling along the nerve. Once this current reaches the end of the nerve, it triggers the release of a neurotransmitter, which then permits the message to be relayed to another cell.

Calcium's role in both muscle contraction and nerve

transmission is especially apparent in the heart. Calcium interacts with potassium and sodium repeatedly in a precisely orchestrated sequence to produce a heartbeat. If your calcium levels are seriously low (which is fairly rare, but it does happen), then your heart's performance can be thrown off, posing a serious danger.

Bowel Binder

In the intestinal tract, calcium can combine—or chelate—with other nutrients and compounds, rendering them unabsorbable. In one recent study, a group of patients receiving approximately 1,000 mg of calcium in their diet and 1,000 mg from supplements excreted twice as much saturated fat (a harmful form of fat) as people receiving normal amounts of calcium only from their diet. These people also experienced a drop in their LDL cholesterol (the "bad" kind) of about 11 percent.

There are also researchers who believe that calcium may have an anti-cancer effect in the colon. It is believed that calcium can bind with cancer-promoting fats and bile acids, which are secreted by the liver. While these bile acids are necessary for proper digestion and assimilation, they can be toxic if produced in large amounts in response to high-fat diets. The calcium binds with these fats and acids, rendering them less toxic and eliminating them more rapidly.

CALCIUM FAST FACTS

Possible Benefits: Osteoporosis, high blood pressure, insomnia, muscle cramps, menstrual cramps, pregnancy-related high blood pressure.

Factors that Deplete Calcium Stores: pregnancy/nursing, lack of exercise, oxalic acid (found in a few foods), high sugar intake, specific metabolic disorders, excessively high-fiber diet, high stress levels.

Supplement Forms: Calcium carbonate, citrate, lactate, citrate-malate, gluconate, and aspartate; dicalcium phosphate; oyster shell, bone meal, and dolomite. Some experts recommend not taking oyster shell or bone meal forms, due to the possibility of lead being present.

Safety Issues: Some experts recommend that calcium supplements not be taken with meals, due to its binding with certain essential minerals such as iron, zinc, copper and manganese, which can deprive the body of these minerals. Also, if you have a kidney disorder or have experienced kidney stones, you need to consult with your doctor before taking supplements. High-calcium intake over short periods is usually considered safe, as the excess is simply excreted.

> *Special Instructions:* When taking calcium supplements, make sure that you take magnesium and vitamin D as well, as both of these are needed for calcium to be properly absorbed and utilized. Most experts also recommend dividing your calcium doses into two separate doses. Avoid taking supplements at the same time as consuming large amounts of wheat bran.

On the Short End

It might come as a surprise to you that most Americans, especially women, are consuming less than the Daily Value (DV) of 1,000 mg of calcium daily. (And many researchers contend that the DV is inadequate anyway.) Women average about 750 mg, and men are just under 1,000 mg. For this reason, most experts recommend taking higher amounts to protect against a deficiency, and ultimately, osteoporosis and other conditions.

Even if you don't develop osteoporosis, invisible damage can take its toll in other ways. For instance, you can develop tiny fractures in your spinal vertebrae, which can cause a condition called dowager's hump, the stooped position that is visible in many elderly people. Moreover, serious and complicated fractures can occur even if you don't have osteoporosis. These are all good reasons to seriously consider calcium.

The Bottom Line

Today, we know more than ever that calcium is not only essential for basic body functions, it is vital in treating and preventing a number of conditions, especially those associated with the musculoskeletal system. Supplements can help promote healthy bones, preventing the often tragic condition of osteoporosis. Calcium can also ensure that muscles (including the heart) are functioning optimally. New research is showing promise for calcium in other areas, including weight loss. So make sure you get your calcium supplements—your body will thank you for it.

18

Grapeseed Extract

YOU HAVE PROBABLY HEARD about the many health benefits of red wine and the studies which have shown that people who live in wine regions live longer. What you may not know is that grapeseed, something available to people living in any region, has amazing antioxidant properties and may be your best defense against the effects of aging. Grapeseed does this, in part, by protecting against cell damage caused by pesticides, food additives and pollution.

Recent studies have shown that air pollution, cigarette smoke, pesticides, contaminated water, and even the food we eat can produce free radicals. Free radicals are unstable or "bad" oxygen molecules that cause damage to other cells. Excess free radicals cause what is called oxidation damage to our bodies. This damage can impair the proper functioning of the immune system, which leads to infections and a hoard of degenerative diseases, including heart disease and cancer. Although not a cure for cancer, antioxidants have been shown to greatly reduce the incidence of all types of cancer. Grapeseed, an excellent source of antioxidants, can be taken to protect cellular DNA from both oxidative damage and cell mutations which can lead to cancer. It also can reduce free radicals and help eliminate the damage they can do.

Until the discovery of grapeseed extract, the best sources of antioxidants were vitamin C, vitamin E and beta carotene. However, these sources are not as powerful as grapeseed and they are used or excreted within a short time of entering the body. Grapeseed, besides exhibiting great antioxidant strength, is an anti-allergenic, antihistamine, and anti-inflammatory. It also strengthens blood vessels, improves skin, and aids in circulation.

The Power of OPCs

The amazing antioxidant power of grapeseed lies in its high concentration of a group of complex substances known as oligomeric proanthocyanidins (OPCs) or procyanidins. OPCs are found in grape seeds and skin, as well as in other blue, red and purple fruits such as plums, blueberries, and cherries. Another good source of OPCs is bark from the maritime pine tree. What can OPCs do for you? The OPCs found in grapeseed act in a variety of biological, pharmacological and therapeutic ways against free radicals and oxidative stress. OPCs are highly effective in part because they neutralize free radicals, but also because they conserve and regenerate vitamins C and E. Vitamin E is a powerful free radical scavenger, but it is quickly used up. OPCs and vitamin C work synergistically to regenerate vitamin E. These three sources then work together to fight off disease.

The Heartening Effects of OPCs

Experimental studies have recently discovered that oxidation of LDL cholesterol is a key factor leading to hardening of the arteries and heart disease. The antioxidant effect of vitamin E and OPCs has been shown to be a potent inhibitor of cholesterol oxidation. OPCs have also been shown to prevent the stickiness of blood platelets that can lead to blood clots and strokes. Patients taking grapeseed extract have reported reduced blood pressure and cholesterol levels. A study published by the American Heart Association showed that six glasses of grape juice were as effective as two glasses of wine in preventing heart disease. This study offers convincing evidence that OPCs from grapes, rather than the alcohol, provide wine's protective benefits to the circulatory system.

OPCs have many other functions. They are one of only a few antioxidant sources that crosses the blood/brain barrier to protect neural tissue. This property may explain why OPCs have been able to help patients with such nerve diseases as multiple sclerosis (MS). MS is a syndrome of progressive destruction and hardening of the myelin sheath that surrounds the nerves. The ability of

GRAPESEED EXTRACT FAST FACTS

Possible Benefits: Grapeseed works as an antioxidant, anti-inflammatory (reduces swelling), antihistamine, and anti-allergenic. It also improves circulation, promotes healing, restores collagen, and strengthens weak blood vessels.

Dietary Sources and Product Forms: OPCs are found in many types of foods, but usually only in extremely small amounts. Some of the best sources are seasonal fruits such as grapes, blueberries, cherries and plums. The are usually found mainly in the peels, skins, or seeds. Food processing and storage is detrimental to OPC availability. You can also buy grapeseed extract in capsule form. There are many producers, so ask your local supplement provider for his/her recommendations. The highest known concentration (95 percent) of the OPC complex is found in grapeseeds, and the second-highest (80–85 percent) in pine bark.

Other names: An important name for the OPC complex is "pycnogenol." This was the name originally given to the complex by Dr. Jacques Masquelier, the first to scientifically discover OPCs and the first to patent their extraction process from the bark of maritime pine trees. "Pycnogenol" is now a trademarked name for OPC products extracted from pine bark.

OPCs to reduce the progressive symptoms of MS is due to their potent antioxidant and anti-allergic qualities. Other diseases associated with aging may also be influenced by OPCs. The ability of OPCs to cross the blood-brain barrier may explain why patients taking an OPC supplement often report improved mental clarity.

Another benefit of OPCs observed by doctors as early as 1950 is anti-inflammatory action. This is produced in part by their antioxidant effect, and also by inhibiting the release and synthesis of compounds that promote inflammation, such as histamine and prostaglandins. OPCs selectively bind to the connective tissue of joints, thus preventing swelling, helping heal damaged tissue, and decreasing pain. OPCs also act as an antihistamine by inhibiting the effect of the enzyme responsible for the production of histamine[histidine decarboxylase]. This effect is enhanced by the ability of OPCs to block another enzyme [hyaluronidase] that facilitates the release of histamine into body tissues.

The antihistamine activity of OPCs also seems to positively affect allergy and ulcer sufferers. OPCs have the ability to strengthen the cell membranes of basophils and mast cells, both of which contain the allergy chemicals. Because the chemicals are not released as easily, over-reaction or hypersensitivity to pollens and food allergens is prevented. Ulcers induced or aggravated by stress are known to be related to excessive secretion of histamine in the stomach lining. OPCs help heal ulcers by reducing histamine secretion and by binding to and protecting connective tissue in mucous membranes. Many who suffer from allergies and/or ulcers have reported significant relief using grapeseed extract.

The Wonders of Anti-Aging OPCs

The OPC constituents in grapeseed also work to combat many of the effects we see as a normal part of the aging process. They accomplish this partly through their ability to enhance immune resistance. OPCs make up one of the most important immune system nutrients to come along in the past fifty years They remain in the body for three full days and are twenty times stronger than vitamin C and fifty times stronger than vitamin E. They are also bioavailable and immediately absorbed from the stomach into the bloodstream. And they are distributed to virtually every organ and tissue. These properties contribute to grapeseed's strength in boosting the immune system. A healthy immune system is vital to reversing the aging process and for providing a long and healthy life. Strong immune systems contribute to capillary strength, increase peripheral circulation, and reduce skin aging and elasticity.

Grapeseed also enhances capillary strength and vascular function, which helps the heart and decreases bruising, edema from injury or trauma, varicose veins, leg swelling and retinopathy. These results come from OPC compounds that have the unique property of strengthening the walls of arteries, veins, and capillaries. New studies show that grapeseed extract is important in helping to prevent heart disease. One study in particular demonstrated that the extract reduced vascular cell damage and secretion of cell adhesion molecules in human endothelial cells—a root cause of many heart disorders typically brought on by age.

By increasing peripheral circulation, OPCs work to improve vision. Clinical studies have shown that antioxidants can halt cataract progression. OPCs have a strong affinity for the portion of the retina that is responsible for visual acuity. They prevent free radical damage and reinforce the collagen structures of the retina. In clinical trials of patients with various types of retinal disease, including macular degeneration, all patients given OPCs showed significant improvement following therapy. Health professionals monitoring the effects of OPCs have reported that it has also helped in the prevention and treatment of glaucoma.

Finally, OPCs help reduce the aging of skin and loss of elasticity. Because of this, grapeseed extract is often used topically in cosmetic preparations. Studies have indicated that OPCs inhibit enzymes such as collagenase, elastase, and hyaluronidase, all of which are involved in the breakdown of structural components of the skin. OPC products help protect the skin from ultraviolet radiation damage that leads to wrinkles and skin cancer. Because it stabilizes collagen and elastin, OPCs can help improve the elasticity and youthfulness of the skin. They also strengthen the connective tissue of the skin and fat chambers. When that connection is broken, the quality of the skin changes. There is speculation that cellulite may actually be a sign of OPC deficiency. is that people taking grapeseed have noticed that it helps tone their skin and reduce cellulite, stretch marks, and old scars—all unwanted signs of aging.

The Bottom Line

Grapeseed extract is a powerful antioxidant which can reduce the damage done by free radicals, strengthen and repair connective tissue, and promote enzyme activity. It can also help moderate allergic and inflammatory responses by reducing histamine production. These actions help fight disease and boost your immune system. If you want to improve your chances against disease, enhance your overall level of health and fight the effects of aging, the OPCs in grapeseed can help you.

19

Micronized Natural Progesterone

HORMONES. IT'S A TOPIC that most women find fearful and confusing. And there's good reason for this—you don't have to look far for contradictory information, a lot of hype (concerning both natural and conventional medicines), and news reports of the terrible side effects associated with hormone replacement therapy (HRT).

In July 2002, the *Journal of the American Medical Association* issued research concluding that long-term use of standard HRT drugs may increase the risk of cardiovascular disease in postmenopausal women. Soon after, the National Institutes of Health announced that it had canceled a major clinical trial involving the use of HRT drugs due to an increased risk of breast cancer and the lack of overall benefit. Both of these events were big news, because literally millions of women across America and elsewhere were or had been taking these drugs (and many

> **THE PEPI TRIAL AND PROGESTERONE**
>
> The first real study to adequately investigate the effectiveness of micronized natural progesterone was the PEPI trial, a multi-centered, placebo-controlled, double-blind study sponsored by the National Institutes of Health. The much-anticipated results from this trial helped answer many questions surrounding menopause and the use of different forms of hormone replacement therapy. In the three-year study of almost 900 women, researchers discovered the following:
>
> - Combining estrogen with progesterone does help protect women against endometrial cancer.
> - Estrogen combined with natural, micronized progesterone provided the best protection of all the combined regimens tested and nearly equal to taking estrogen alone.
> - The study also discovered that women taking hormones (especially natural progesterone) after menopause gained less weight than women taking no hormones at all.

still are). For the past forty years, HRT has been used in medicine to treat the discomforts of menopause and prevent diseases—such as cardiovascular disease and osteoporosis—associated with aging women.

Natural Hormones vs. Synthetic Hormones

Before we talk about natural progesterone and (specifically micronized progesterone), perhaps we should define "progesterone" regarding HRT use. The progesterone-like compounds prescribed by doctors for use in conventional HRT, typically called "progestins" and which go by the name Provera (or some other generic name), are a synthetic drug that is chemically similar, but not identical, to your own progesterone. Truly, these progestins are not hormones at all, but rather they are drugs that are synthesized to be chemically similar to real progesterone. Likewise, the "estrogen" that is prescribed to women as part of HRT, typically under the product name Premarin, is a synthesized drug based on the estrogen of pregnant horses. It is not chemically identical to a woman's estrogen; rather it is identical to a horse's estrogen.

Now let's talk about the natural forms of progesterone. Unlike most of the supplements covered in this book, the products we'll cover in this chapter are available only by prescription or through compounding pharmacies (as opposed to the more ubiquitous health food stores, regular pharmacies, and the like). But they are natural products in that they are produced to be structurally and chemically identical to your own hormones. And many doctors who have long had doubts about conventional HRT treatment strongly endorse these natural versions of progesterone.

As mentioned before, the natural forms of progesterone

that are recommended are identical to your own progesterone, and are usually synthesized from compounds taken from soybeans or wild yam. But they aren't available from your local health food store. They are only available through prescription from a licensed medical doctor or through compounding pharmacies. While there are still many doctors who aren't familiar with the natural forms of progesterone, the number is growing who are educating themselves to their benefits (especially after the announcements from the National Institutes of Health).

Natural Progesterone

The natural progesterone products now available are made up of natural compounds and structured to be an exact replica of human progesterone. The most commonly used progesterones are nonproprietary products, usually going by the name "micronized" progesterone or progesterone USP, that are available through compounding pharmacies and in a variety of dosages. Or the patented versions, called Prometrium (capsules) or Crinone (vaginal cream), are available through regular pharmacies.

There is much discussion as to which form—the capsules or vaginal creams—are best. Some experts, such as Uzzi Reiss, M.D., advocate the use of capsules as generally being most effective. He says, however, that the creams may be the best route for certain individuals, depending on their condition and needs. You should consult with your doctor concerning which form will work best for you.

Heart-Healthy Progesterone

When it comes to the issues of hormones, menopause and the like, women tend to focus on the more high-profile issue of breast cancer. Yet heart disease has been the number one killer of women for decades. Roughly 240,000 women die from heart-related ailments every year, a number nearly five times that of breast cancer deaths.

It is well-known that estradiol and the standard chemicalized estrogen replacement Premarin have powerful heart-protecting effects. They can increase the levels of "good" cholesterol and lower the levels of "bad" cholesterol, improve coronary artery dilation, and reduce the formation of arterial plaque.

However, it is also well-known that if progestins, the synthetic form of progesterone found in standard HRT medications, are combined with the estradiol/Premarin, these heart-protective effects are lost. The progestin cancels them out and increases the risk of heart disease. In short, researchers have discovered that progestins do two things:

1. They cancel the protective effects of estradiol, and

2. It promotes the constriction of the coronary arteries to a significant degree beyond that of the artery constricting chemical alone.

In simple terms, the research regarding all of the latest

progestin drugs shows that they result in more oxidative damage to arteries, more arterial plaque, more constricted arteries, and ultimately, more heart disease. The findings clearly explain why researchers concluded recently that the standard hormone replacement therapy doesn't protect you from cardiovascular disease. The reason is not because of the estrogen component, but because of the negative effect of the progestin.

Conversely, the research on natural progesterone supplements show that it does not hinder the benefits of estrogen on the heart. This should come as no surprise—if it had a negative effect, then pregnancy would be a serious risk-factor for a heart attack. That's when a woman's progesterone levels rise dramatically. But it is well-known that this simply is not the case.

The Breast Cancer Connection

Various studies have shown that progesterone (the natural kind) significantly decreases the risk of breast cancer and dramatically improves the prognosis of women who develop breast cancer. Here are some of the ways it does this:

- It enhances a protective gene system (known as P53), which slows down another gene system (BCL2) that promotes the development of cancer.

- It decreases the gene survivin, which acts in a similar manner to the cancer-causing system BCL2.

PROGESTERONE FAST FACTS

Product Availability: Capsules, vaginal creams/gels, skin creams, sublingual drops

Possible Benefits: Decreased hot flashes and night sweating, reduced risk of osteoporosis, heart disease, Alzheimer's disease, decreased water retention, healthy weight maintenance, increased sexual interest, improved moods and state of mind, increased stamina, improved sleep, healthier skin, decreased risk of cancer, prevention of endometrial hyperplasia (tissue overgrowth within the endometrium), reversing secondary amenorrhea

Possible Side Effects/Cautions: It is best to take estrogen in conjunction with natural progesterone. For this purpose, consult with your doctor and encourage him or her to customize a regimen that best works for you. Signs of excess progesterone replacement may include drowsiness, dizziness, heaviness of the fingers, hands or feet. A very few women may experience other symptoms, including anxiety, poor sleep, retaining of water, hot flashes, depression, and increased weight gain.

Individuals with allergies to peanuts should avoid the product Prometrium, as it contains peanut oil. In this case, it may be best to try the generic products available through a compounding pharmacy.

> *Special Instructions:* Because each woman is an individual and different in her needs, it is wise to insist on a program that can be adjusted in terms of dosage amounts, times and which form is taken. Also, generally speaking, best results are achieved if progesterone is taken with natural estrogen. If your doctor is not familiar with natural estrogen and progesterone, talk to him or her about both natural estrogen and progesterone, and explain that you would like to consider them as options for your hormone program. For more information, see *Natural Hormone Balance for Women,* by Uzzi Reiss, M.D., and *What Your Doctor May Not Tell You About Breast Cancer,* by John R. Lee, M.D.

- It prevents the body's cells from dividing and proliferating excessively in tissues of the breast and uterus.

- It normalizes the process of apoptosis, which is the mechanism that allows cells to commit "suicide." Apoptosis deters cells form transforming into harmful forms due to chemical reactions in the body.

- It reduces the ability of breast cancer cells to metastasize (spread to other parts of the body).

Natural Progesterone and the Brain

We know that estrogen in proper amounts is helpful for optimum brain function. Many doctors have reported the remarkable ability of estrogen supplements to transform a woman low in estrogen within just a matter of hours. These patients go from having a veritable case of "brain fog" to enjoying a clear mind and improved mental awareness.

Your own progesterone also aids the brain. It calms, relaxes and protects the nervous system. It helps you get adequate sleep, and improves the quality of sleep. It can also play an important role in decreasing feelings of anxiety, depression and related mood swings.

Contrasting this, the synthetic progestins can actually damage nerve cells, and overexcite the nervous sytem. They have been shown to increase anxiety, nervousness and adversely affect sleep. For these reasons, the use of natural progesterone rather than progestins is advisable.

The Osteoporosis Link

Regarding the topic of osteoporosis and bone health, progesterone is your best friend. Working together with estrogen, progesterone initiates the growth of new bone tissue and delays the loss of "old" bone tissue.

Despite popular opinion otherwise, some researchers feel that progesterone is at least as important, if not more, than estrogen when it comes to increasing bone mass, strengthening bone tissue and preventing the onset of osteoporosis. Another important note is that some forms of injectable progestins used mainly for birth control have been shown to decrease bone density in young women, creating in them a greater risk for osteoporosis later in life.

Natural progesterone benefits the body in other ways, including the following:

- It's a natural diuretic, reducing the amount of water retention.

- It may minimize the discomforts of PMS and menstruation.

- It improves the breakdown of fat into energy.

- It prevents endometrial hyperplasia (tissue overgrowth) when used with estrogen.

- It can help reverse secondary amenorrhea (abnormal stopping of period in a woman who otherwise should be menstruating).

- It can reduce the craving for simple carbohydrates, especially "sweets."

- It reduces breast tenderness and pain.

> **WILD YAM: THE "OTHER" NATURAL PROGESTERONE**
>
> When searching for a natural progesterone product, especially creams, be aware that there are products that advertise themselves as "natural progesterone" that are different from micronized natural progesterone. These products are usually extracts of Mexican wild yam, which has demonstrated effects similar to progesterone, but not exactly. And, it is significantly weaker in its action. The truth is, wild yam does contain compounds from which natural progesterone is made, but your body cannot convert them into progesterone when you eat them. While it does possess some benefit, and there is some research backing its abilities, understand that it is different from micronized progesterone both in its chemical structure and its actions.

What About Natural Estrogen?

Just as there are now natural forms of progesterone, you can find natural estrogen; that is, estrogen that has been produced to be an identical match to the estrogen found in the human body as opposed to the standard HRT drugs, such as Premarin, that were only similar. These products can be obtained in a micronized form from pharmacies or through a prescription by your doctor. Many doctors are lauding the effects of natural estrogen, especially when used in conjunction with natural progesterone. There a few commonly used estrogen products, including Tri-Est and Estrace. Tri-Est is a combination of the three estrogen forms naturally found in the body, estriol (80 percent), estradiol and estrone (each 10 percent). While there is still little research on natural estrogen, it is FDA approved and there are several notable doctors, including John Lee, M.D. and Uzzi Reiss, M.D., that highly endorse its use. Like natural progesterone products, natural estrogen is available through a prescription by your doctor and/or through a compounding pharmacy.

One important thing to remember about estrogen is that it requires progesterone to work and not become a hazard to the body. The following is a list of potential dividends resulting from using natural estrogen in hormone replacement therapy, usually in conjunction with natural progesterone:

- Improved control of emotions and thinking
- Increased stamina and energy
- Better-quality sleep
- Healthier skin
- Increased interest in sex
- More ease in maintaining a healthy weight
- Breasts that are more full
- Elimination of hot flashes/night sweats
- Reduced risk of heart disease
- Reduced risk of osteoporosis
- Reduced risk of Alzheimer's disease

The Bottom Line

For many years, estrogen was considered the dominant and most important of the female hormones. Now we understand that progesterone is just as vital in the health of every woman. More importantly, we know that micronized natural progesterone offers the same benefits (sometimes even better) and reduced side effects as the synthetic drug versions offered in standard HRT programs. In a time when millions of women are confused and fearful of hormone replacement, natural progesterone offers a incredible option that will invariably improve the life of the woman taking it.

20

"Green" and "Phyto" Foods

YOU MAY ASK YOURSELF, "What exactly are 'green' or 'phyto' foods?" It's a good question. Phyto simply means "plant," so phytonutrient products contain nutrients derived from plants. The term "green foods" is used for the same type of products since most of the ingredients are substances derived from plants (many of them being green, of course).

Each of these nutrients is thought to have some sort of health benefit. Some may help digestion or reduce inflammation, while others fight chronic pain or reduce cholesterol levels. Others may improve the functioning of cells or protect from free radicals.

While most vegetables and fruits have some nutritional value, and are preferred dietary components over synthetic processed foods, there are other "green" foods—which include families of algae, cereal grasses and legumes—that

WHAT THE LABELS AREN'T TELLING US

It's somewhat difficult to determine just by looking at a product's label whether you're getting a substantial amount of a phytonutrient or just a smidgen. Since there is no standardization of such products, and all of them vary in their ingredients, you can count on inconsistency between products.

Still, there are steps you can take to ensure that you are getting what you paid for. First, don't assume that the most expensive product is the best. Some reviewers have found that some of the best products have also been the cheapest. Also, look for labels that provide specific ingredients, especially ones that indicate they are standardized extracts. If it just says "broccoli," then you are paying a top-dollar price for some freeze-dried broccoli instead of the concentrated extract. It's no guarantee, but it does suggest some degree of quality control. Another step to consider is to buy a product from a major manufacturer or major store brand, who has more to lose if it's revealed that a product doesn't deliver on its promises.

An additional factor to consider when looking for green food products is to see which extract(s) you want the most of, and then seek out a product that has significant amounts of that particular substance.

possess particular dietary value. Why? There are several reasons. First, these phyto-foods usually contain high levels of chlorophyll, a pigment responsible for the plants' green color and the ability to employ sunlight and utilize minerals from the soil to make starches, fats, proteins, vitamins and other substances a plant requires from life. Many experts believe that chlorophyll can be a potent health-promoting substance. Second, these plants are full of most of the other basic nutrients a human body requires for optimal health; these include minerals, vitamins, bioflavonoids, antioxidants, proteins, amino acids, essential fatty acids, enzymes and coenzymes, and fiber, among others. Third, it is only through these plants that the human body can obtain some of the previously listed nutrients; that is, these green foods are essential for certain body processes and structures. Finally, these foods are not only necessary for maintaining the various body systems and processes, but can also play a key role in aggressively combatting the many diseases and disorders the human body is susceptible to.

The notion that certain foods, in this case "green" foods, provide the body with essential nutrients may raise the question of whether or not we consume enough of these foods in our daily diet. For the majority of Americans, the answer is an overwhelming "no." This may explain the emergence of green food or green drink products that can be prepared easily and consumed regularly. What are in these products? Though the ingredients of these products may vary somewhat, most contain a core group that sup-

GREEN FOODS FAST FACTS

Possible Benefits: Nutrient deficiencies, cancer, stroke, heart disease, macular degeneration, overall health improvement

Possible Product Names: Any product with the term "green" or "phyto" in the title, such as green food, green drink, phytonutrients, phyto-food; Individual names: carotenes, carotenoids, proanthocyanidins, anthocyanins, isoflavones, lycopene, lutein, zeaxanthin, and many others.

Special Instructions: Many experts recommend taking green food products with meals.

Food Sources: Blueberries, strawberries, green tea, oranges, red onion, cabbage, broccoli, carrot, kale, pumpkin, squash, garlic, onion, tomatoes, spinach, grapefruit, lemons, limes, red and green peppers, cayenne peppers, apricots, peaches, beets, wheat grass, barley grass, kelp, spirulina, chlorella, and many other vegetables, fruits, grasses and herbs

Safety Issues: Do not consider green foods as a replacement for a healthful diet. Neglecting proper dietary habits can lead to serious nutrient deficiencies and/or health conditions.

ply a valuable assembly of phytonutrients. For instance, one product currently available contains lutein, lycopene, wheat grass, spirulina, beta carotene, bioflavonoids, quercetin, cayenne pepper, red cabbage extract, garlic extract, barley grass extract, grape seed extract, green tea extract, zeaxanthin, elderberry extract, broccoli extract, and rosemary.

And what are these phyto-foods purported to do? Primarily, their best asset is that of promoting overall good health and in disease prevention. But many consumers look at their green food capsules or drinks as actual disease fighters—to reverse macular degeneration, stimulate a sluggish thyroid, improve digestion problems, prevent cancer, enhance immune function, and many more.

The idea of putting so many of these substances in one product is that in theory, all of the specific ingredients has one or more health benefits, so potentially the product can provide the body with a variety of protective benefits and encourage an improved state of health.

Primary Color Groups of "Phyto-Foods"

One way that health-savvy individuals identify with foods is by their color. A vegetable or fruit's color can indicate what sort of nutrients it contains, and thereby suggest how it may be beneficial for the body. The following subsections break down the various color groups among the vegetables, fruits and other plants, and which nutrients are most prominently found in them.

Greens

The "green" group of "phyto-foods" include spirulina, chlorella, kelp, blue-green algae, dulce, wheat grass, barley grass, alfalfa, soy extracts, broccoli, spinach, parsley, lime, celery, kale, cabbage, kamut grass, rice grass, oat grass (and other grasses).

Greens are excellent sources of chlorophyll, B vitamins, vitamin C, antioxidants (like vitamins E and A, selenium), carotenoids, beta carotene, calcium, iron, zinc, indoles, GLA, vegetable protein and other nutrients.

Reds, Yellows, Oranges

This group includes tomato, cranberry, cayenne, red and yellow bell pepper, orange juice, carrot, Norwegian kelp, grapefruit, pineapple, brown rice, papaya, apricot, and squash.

Reds provide various carotenes, vitamin C, capsaicin, phytofuene, phtoene, and licopenes. The yellow and orange group provides rich sources of vitamin C, carotenoids, various carotenes, iodine, phytofluene and phytoene, pectin, fiber and protein digestive aids.

Blue/Purple

This group includes black cherry, grapeskin extract, beet juice, and elderberry. This group is known especially for its antioxidant content, including that of proanthocyanidins, and for its high bioflavonoid content. These foods also provide various phenols and ellagic acid.

White

This group includes apple pectin, garlic, and onion. These foods are known for its allium and allyl sulfide content, and are high in fiber and pectin.

Herbs

The herbal group, which would consist mainly of "green" phyto-foods, includes echinacea, milk thistle, *Ginkgo biloba*, green tea extract, ginger, hawthorn, *Garcinia cambogia*, ginseng, *Gymnema sylvestre*, licorice, Atlantic kelp, astragalus, stevia, horsetail, and others.

These herbs are the most common found in "green food" products mainly for their powerful nutritional content and therapeutic capabilities. They are used for a wide variety of purposes, from supporting and stimulating the immune system, to promoting a strong vascular system, to normalizing glandular function. The majority of these particular herbs are also high in essential vitamins, minerals and other nutrients.

Bee Products

These include bee pollen, royal jelly, propolis and honey. Though not all bee products are technically plant related, they are recognized as an excellent source of a wide variety of essential nutrients, including vitamins, trace minerals, enzymes, coenzymes, amino acids, essential fatty acids, and more. Therefore, they are often included in green food products.

AFTER TABLETS AND CAPSULES, WHAT ELSE?

There are many different green food products, with the majority of them being capsules and/or tablets. But there are other forms of green foods that just might appeal to you:

Powders, Granules and Flakes: For a quick breakfast, snack, or after-meal treat, mix sea green powders, granules or flakes, or cereal grasses with fruit or vegetable juices, blend well, and drink (since green foods are usually so digestible, this will provide a quick energy "kick"). Granules and flakes, and cereal grasses can be also add a touch of excitement to salads or cooked grains.

Juicing: Though technically not a supplement, juicing is a very popular way of getting your green food fix, mainly due to the fact that juice is one of the easiest forms of food for the body to assimilate. This means that within minutes, the vitamins, minerals, enzymes and other phytonutrients contained in the juice are being assimilated by the body. Unlike digesting solid foods, the body requires little energy to metabolize juices.

Different types of juices can also have different functions. For instance, fruit juices typically act as cleansers and vegetable juices act as tonics and builders. Juice fasts are typically done with fruit juices, since they are

> effective cleansers. Vegetable juices are used to supplement fruit juice fasts, supplying the body with needed proteins while the body detoxifies.
>
> Juicing can also have other benefits. Taking juice between meals can effectively cut down on cravings for unhealthy or unnecessary foods; this can especially be effective for children or those trying to lose weight. Also, because of their high nutritional content, juices can replace "heavy" foods that we may normally eat at meals. This cuts down substantially on fat and cholesterol intake, and allows the body to avoid wasting energy on metabolizing unnecessary foods.

The Bottom Line

Although there is little research on green food or phytonutrient combination products, there is plenty of research on many of the individual ingredients that may make up these products. Potentially, these concentrated forms of various health-promoting nutrients can be very beneficial to the body, especially in the areas of general health and disease prevention. As a supplement, there is little to suggest that a green food supplement can hurt you (though it is always wise to follow the recommendations on the label and to consult with your doctor). On the other hand, it is imperative that you not consider these products as a replacement for a well-rounded diet. However, because it is increasingly more difficult to get all the nutrients necessary for excellent health, they are an excellent choice to supplement and enhance our dietary habits.

21

Other Essential Supplements

So MAYBE YOU'VE READ through the entire book and found that you'd like to research additional supplements. Or maybe the top twenty we've focused on aren't quite what you're looking for. Well you're in luck. We have included here a list of additional supplements that either have shown promise but are lacking the scientific backing, or are proven but more narrow in their scope of health benefits. Who knows? Maybe one or more of these will make it to the top twenty in the next edition of *20 Essential Supplements*!

Rhodiola: The root of this plant has been used for centuries in China, Serbia and the Ukraine for a variety of reasons. Current research shows promising potential for rhodiola in the areas of increasing energy, fighting fatigue, improving mental function and promoting heart health, among others. This is a recently emerging supplement in the United States and has been received with much excitement.

Transfer Factor: This exciting compound is found in colostrum (the mother's first milk) and transfers immune information to the offspring. Transfer factors have been studied and found to be effective at preventing and fighting infections of various kinds. At present, one company—4Life Research—holds the patent to producing transfer factor products.

Lycopene: This carotenoid, which is found principally in tomatoes and is the most widely consumed carotenoid in America, has shown to be an effective antioxidant and anticancer agent. Research indicates that it may reduce the risk of prostate cancer, breast cancer and different skin cancers.

Glucosamine: For several years, glucosamine has been studied and shown to be effective in fighting the effects of joint conditions such as osteoarthritis. It helps prevent the loss of joint tissue and reduces pain and inflammation.

Conjugated Linoleic Acid: Research shows that this beneficial fat can aid the body in reducing unwanted body fat while simultaneously increasing muscle. And because CLA is becoming increasingly difficult to receive through the typical diet, supplementation may be the ideal way to get this impressive fatty acid.

Ginkgo: This popular herbal product has long been known to help with problems related to poor circulation. Research shows it can help increase blood flow to the brain, thereby improving mental function. It can also help with male erectile dysfunction.

Hyperimmune Egg: This product is derived from eggs that come from chickens exposed to various diseases. Thus, the egg carries immune information that can help the body create antibodies to those diseases without actually being exposed to the disease. There is promising research on immune egg products.

Guggul: This resin from the mukul tree is widely used in Ayurvedic medicine to treat arthritis, lower high blood pressure and moderate triglyceride levels. Western science has backed these uses as well as others.

Bilberry: This remarkable berry, also known as European blueberry, has been shown to aid in both preventing and reversing a number of eye-related ailments, including glaucoma. It also appears to help with vascular problems, such as decreased circulation to the extremities, and may possess anticancer properties.

Ashwagandha: This Ayurvedic herb has been widely used as a general tonic. Recent investigation shows it may help with arthritic symptoms, improved energy levels and increased sexual performance.

Bee Products: These include bee pollen, propolis, royal jelly and honey. They are widely used to treat allergies, promote increased energy and stamina, boost immune function and act as a superior source of various vitamins, minerals, enzymes and other helpful nutrients.

MSM: Methylsulfonylmethane (MSM) is a form of sulfur that is used to produce crucial enzymes, antibodies, glutathione (the body's principal antioxidant) and connective tissue such as cartilage, collagen and skin. It is also critical for the production and proper use of amino acids. Research shows that MSM supplementation can help with a variety of ailments, including severe allergies, asthma and arthritis.

St. John's Wort: This wonder herb took the health world by storm a few years back as an effective treatment for mild to moderate depression. It is also effective in relieving related conditions such as anxiety and sleep dysfunction. There are adverse interactions with some prescription drugs, so make sure to consult with your physician before taking it.

Valerian/Passionflower: Both of these herbs, which are often found in combination with one another, are excellent options for treating nervous and emotional problems such as anxiety, stress, and insomnia and other sleep disorders.

Hawthorn: This herb, which has widely used in Europe for decades, is an excellent promoter of heart health. Studies show it can help fight and prevent various forms of heart disease. There is also research indicating that it can aid in normalizing sleep patterns and related sleep dysfunction.

Milk Thistle Extract: Milk thistle and its principal compound, silymarin, have dozens of studies and literally thousands of health professionals touting their ability to both halt damage to the liver and stimulate the regeneration of liver cells. Milk thistle extract is an excellent option for those with even severe liver damage. It also is used to treat mild digestive problems.

Seroctin: This is a very new product comprised of certain plant compounds that have a beneficial effect on mood and emotional health, probably through their action on serotonin production. Research indicates that seroctin may also improve sexual function and increase libido.

Grapefruit Seed Extract: This relatively new supplement was principally used for external purposes to treat such problems as nail fungus, infections, psoriasis and the like. Research shows that grapefruit seed possesses potent antimicrobial capabilities. It has been shown to both directly and indirectly counter viruses, fungi, bacteria and yeast. Supplements are now available for internal use, especially for fighting *Candida albicans* and other chronic infections.

L-arginine: This amino acid has been proven to help fight against sexual dysfunction in men, particularly with maintaining an erection. It also stimulates the production of growth hormone, which is instrumental in shedding fat and building muscle. It is also used medically to promote wound healing in patients after surgery or for those suffering from severe burns.

Lipoic Acid: This is a powerful antioxidant that can protect the body from various conditions. It has been widely used in Europe to fight the effects of diabetes, and research here shows it offers a variety of benefits, from improving physical endurance to reducing the effects of stroke to possibly protecting from heart disease.

Selected References

Abdalla et al. 1985. Prevention of bone mineral loss in postmenopausal women by norethisterone. Obstet Gynecol 66:789–92.

Albert, A. et al. Efficacy and safety of a phytoestrogen preparation derived from Glycine max (L.) Merr in . . . Phytomedicine March, 2002; 9(2): 85–92.

Balch, Phyllis, Balch, James. Prescription for Nutritional Healing. Avery, New York: 2000.

Bernard et al. 2001. Antiproliferative and antiapoptotic effects of crel may occur within the same cells via the up-regulation of manganese superoxide dismutase. Cancer Research 15:61(6):2656–64.

Bisignano, G. et al. On the in-vitro antimicrobial activity of oleuropein and hydroxytyrosol. J Pharm Pharmacol. August, 1999; 51(8): 971–4.

Bordia et al. 1998. Effect of garlic (Allium sativa) on blood lipids, blood sugar, fibrinogen and fibrinolytic activity in patients with coronary artery disease. Prostaglandins Leukot Essent Fatty Acids 58(4):257–63.

Bracke et al. 1999. Influence of tangeretin on tamoxifen's therapeutic benefit in mammary cancer. J Natl Cancer Inst 91:354–359.

Braeckman, J. Current Therapeutic Research, 55 (1994): 776–85.

Brief, et al. 2001. Use of glucosamine and chondroitin sulfate in the management of osteoarthritis. J Am Acad Orthop Surg 9(2):71–8.

Castillo et al. 2000. Antioxidant activity and radioprotective effects against chromosomal damage induced in vivo by X-rays of flavan-3-ols (Procyanidins) from grape seeds (Vitis vinifera): Comparative study versus other phenolic and organic compounds. J Agric Food Chem 48(5):1738–45.

Champault, G., et al. British Journal of Clinical Pharmacology, 18(1984): 461–62.

Cusi et al. 2001. Vanadyl sulfate improves hepatic and muscle insulin sensitivity in type II diabetes. Journal of Clinical Endocrinology Metabolism 86(3):1410–7.

D.T. Chu et al., Chinese Journal of Oncology, 16(3) (1994): 167–71.

Davidson et al. 1997. Effects of docosahexaenoic acid on serum lipoproteins in patients with combined hyperlipidemia: A randomized, double-blind, placebo-controlled trial. J Am Coll Nutr 16(3):236–43.

Douglas, et al. Vitamin C for preventing and treating the common cold. Cochrane Database System Review; 2002, 3(2):CD000980.

Elkins, Rita. Miracle Sugars. Woodland Publishing; Pleasant Grove, Utah, 2002.

Erden, M. and A. Kahraman. 2000. The protective effect of flavonol quercitin against ultraviolet a induced oxidative stress in rats. Toxicology 23:154(1–3):21–9.

Fletcher, R., Fairfield, K. Vitamins for chronic disease prevention in adults: clinical applications. JAMA. June 2002: 287(23): 3127-9.

Fortes et al. 1998. The effect of zinc and vitamin A supplementation on immune response in an older population. Journal of American Geriatric Society 46(1):19–26.

Fruhbeck, G. 1996. Dietary fiber and coronary heart disease prevention. JAMA. 26:275(24):1883.

Gerber, G. 2000. Saw palmetto for the treatment of men with lower urinary tract symptoms. J Urol 163(5):1408–12.

Goss et al. 2001. Effect of potassium phosphate supplementation on perceptual and physiological responses to maximal graded exercise. International Journal of Sports Nutrition and Exercise Metabolism 11(1):53–62.

Greeson et al. 2001. St. John's wort (Hypericum perforatum): a review of the current pharmacological, toxicological, and clinical literature. Psychopharmacology (Berl) 153(4):402–14.

Haisraeli-Shalish et al. 1996. Recurrent aphthous stomatitis and thiamin deficiency. Oral Surgery Oral Medicine Oral Pathol and Oral Radiology Endodontics 82(6):634–6.

Hughes-Fulford et al. 2001. Fatty acid regulates gene expression and growth of human prostate cancer PC-3 cells. Carcinogenesis 22(5):701–7.

Isolauri et al. 2001. Probiotics in human disease. Am J Clin Nutr 73(6 Part 2):1142S–6S.

Jan.1998.

Kaikkonen et al. 1997. Effect of oral coenzyme Q10 on the oxidation resistance of human VLDL + LDL fraction: absorption and antioxidative properties of oil and granule-based preparations. Free Radic Biol Med 22:1195–1202.

Kamei, et al. 2000. The effect of a traditional Chinese prescription for a case of lung carcinoma. Journal of Alternative and Complementary Medicine Dec. 6(6): 557–9.

Kh, et al. 2000. Effect of oral magnesium supplementation on blood pressure, platelet aggregation and calcium handling in deoxycorticosterone acetate induced hypertension in rats. Journal of Hypertension 8(7):919-26.

Kim, et al. 1996. Antiproliferative effects of low-dose micronized progesterone. Fertility and Sterility 65(2):323–331.

Selected References

Kuroda, et al. 1999. Antimutagenic and anticarcinogenic activity of tea polyphenols. Mutat Res 436(1):69–97.

Lamb, et al. 1999. Dietary copper supplementation reduces atherosclerosis in the cholesterol-fed rabbit. Atherosclerosis 146(1):33-43.

Lieberman, Shari and Bruning, Nancy. The Real Vitamin and Mineral Book, 2nd Ed. Avery, Garden City, New York: 1997.

Lucock, M. and I. Daskalakis. 2000. New perspectives on folate status: a differential role for the vitamin in cardiovascular disease, birth defects and other conditions. British Journal of Biomedicine and Science 57(3):254–60.

Malesky, Gale, and editors of Prevention Health Books. Nature's Medicines. Rodale Press, Inc. Emmaus, Pennsylvania. 1999.

Melchart et al. 1998. Echinacea: Clinical trial re: rhinovirus. Archives of Family Medicine. Nov–Dec.

Mindell, Earl. Earl Mindell's Supplement Bible. Fireside, New York: 1998.

Mondoa, Emil. I. Sugars that Heal. Ballantine Books, 2001.

Morisco et al. 1993. Effect of coenzyme Q10 in patients with congestive heart failure: a long-term multicenter randomized study. Clin Invest 71:S134–36.

Murray, Michael. "Fighting cancer with a cup, or more, of green tea." Better Nutrition

Ng, S.Y. 1999. Hair calcium and magnesium levels in patients with fibromyalgia: a case center study. Journal of Manipulative Physiological Therapy 2(9):586–93.

PDR for Herbal Medicines, 2nd Edition. Montavale, NY: Medical Economics Company, 2000.

Pierce, Andrea. Practical Guide to Natural Medicines. Stonesong Press, Inc. New York, NY. 1999.

Polidori et al. 2001. Plasma vitamin C levels are decreased and correlated with brain damage in patients with intracranial hemorrhage or head trauma. Stroke 32(4):898–902.

Q. Guo et al., Chung-Kuo Chung His I Chieh Ho Tsa Chih, 15(8) (1995):483–85.

Qureshi, M.A., R.A., Ali. "Spirulina platensis exposure enhances macrophage phagocytic function in cats." Immunopharmacol Immunotoxicol. 1996 Aug., (18) 457–463.

Reavley, Nicola. New Encyclopedia of Vitamins, Minerals, Supplements, and Herbs. M.Evans and Company, Inc. New York 1998.

Reiss, Uzzi. Natural Hormone Balance. Pocket Books; New York: 2001.

Seibel, Machelle. The Soy Solution for Menopause. Fireside, New York: 2002.

Shearer, M. 2000. Role of vitamin K and Gla proteins in the pathophysiology of osteoporosis and vascular calcification. Current Opinions in Clinical Nutritional Metabolism Care 3(6):433–8.

Shimizu, S. 1999. Pantothenic acid. Nippon Rinsho 7(10):2218–22.

Shults C.W., et al. Effects of coenzyme Q10 in early Parkinson disease: evidence of slowing of the functional decline. Archives of Neurology. October, 2002; 59(10):1523.

So, et al. 1996. Inhibition of human breast cancer cell proliferation and delay of mammary tumorigenesis by flavonoids and citrus juices. Nutr Cancer 26:167–181.

Sone, H. 2000. Characteristics of the biotin enhancement of glucose-induced insulin release in pancreatic islets of the rat. Bioscience Biotechnology Biochemistry 64(3):550–4.

Soulimani, et al. 1997. Behavioural effects of Passiflora incarnata L. and its indole alkaloid and flavonoid derivatives and maltol in the mouse. J Ethnopharmacol 57(1):11–20.

Sun, et al. 2000. Effects of Ginkgo biloba extract on somatosensory evoked potential, nitric oxide levels in serum and brain tissue in rats with cerebral vasospasm after subarachnoid hemorrhage. Clin Hemorheol Microcirculation 23(2–4):139–44.

Thys-Jacobs, et al. 1998. Calcium carbonate and the premenstrual syndrome: effects on premenstrual and menstrual symptoms. American Journal of Obstetrics and Gynecology 179(2):444–452.

Tichy, J. and J. Novak. 2000. Detection of antimicrobials in bee products with activity against viridans streptococci. J Altern Complement Med 6(5):383–9.

Turner, Lisa. "Energy in a Glass: Green Foods." Let's Live, Nov. 1997, 74.

Tyler, Varro. The Honest Herbal. (Binghamton, NY: Hawthorn Press/Pharmaceutical Products Press, 1993).

Vitamin Cures. Rodale; Emmaus, Pennsylvania: 2002.

Wacker, A. and W. Hilbig, Planta Medica, 33 (1978): 89–102.

Weil, Andrew. Eating Right for Optimum Health. Random House, New York: 2000.

Wood et al. 2000. Beta-carotene and selenium supplementation enhances immune response in aged humans. Integrative Medicine 21:2(2):85–92.

Wyatt et al. 1999. Efficacy of vitamin B-6 in the treatment of premenstrual syndrome: systematic review. British Medical Journal 22:318(7195): 1375–81.

Index

acidophilus (see "probiotics")
adaptogen
    astragalus as 87
American Medical Association
    19–20
allergies 36, 137, 210
antibiotics
    problems with 79–82, 153
anxiety 210
arthritis, 209, 210
    rheumatoid 36, 44, 47–48,
        60–61, 99
    osteoarthritis 44, 47–48, 208
    pantothenic acid and 60–61
asthma 36, 137
ashwagandha 209
Astragalus 87–92
    immunity and 88–90
    heart health and 91
autism 55
bacteria
    probiotic (beneficial) 77–86
bee products 210

benign prostatic hyperplasia
    (BPH) 161–62
beri-beri 61
Beta carotene 27, 107–116
    vision and 110
    immunity and 110–11
    cancer and 113–115
    heart disease and 116
    guidelines for 114–15
bifidobacteria (see "probiotics")
bilberry 209
bioflavonoids 27–28
biotin 65–66
Calcium 30, 167–74
    osteoporosis and 168–70
    supplement forms 169
    muscle/nerve function and
        170–71
    harmful fats and 171
    deficiency of 173
cancer 57, 58–59
    breast 44, 188–90
    colon 44

glyconutrients and 100–101
beta carotene and 113–15
fiber and 119, 121
green tea and 128–29
natural progesterone and 188–90
candida 79, 104, 211
carpal tunnel syndrome 54
cataracts 36
Chinese medicine 87
chlorophyll 199
cholesterol 47, 128–29, 135, 156, 171
chromium 31
chronic fatigue syndrome 74, 90, 101–04,
coenzyme A 60
Coenzyme Q10 133–37
   deficiency of 134–35
   heart disease and 134–35
   Parkinson's disease and 135
cold, common 36, 40–41
   echinacea and 74
   astragalus and 90
   olive leaf and 156–57
conjugated linoleic acid (CLA) 208
constipation
   fiber and 120
copper 31
Coxsackie B virus 91
depression 49, 53, 143, 191, 210, 211
dermatitis 44
diabetes 54, 212
   biotin and 65–66
   fiber and 119, 120
   olive leaf and 158–59
"die-off" effect 159
dietary reference intake (DRI) 14
Dietary Supplement Health and Education Act 10–11
   and dietary supplements 10
docosahexaenoic acid (DHA) 45–46
Echinacea 69–75
   history of 70–71
   immune function and 71–75

eicosapentaenoic acid (EPA) 45–46
energy 41–42, 60, 61–63, 134–35, 159–60
   B vitamins and 51–67
Essential fatty acids (EFAs) 43–50
   Innuit Eskimos and 43–44
   heart disease and 47
   arthritis and 47–48
   cancer and 49
   Crohn's disease and 49
   depression and 49
estrogen 140–43, 193–94
Fiber 117–24
   insoluble/soluble 117–19

fibromyalgia 104
fish oil (see essential fatty acids)
flaxseed 44

Index

flu 36, 40–41, 130
    echinacea and 74
    astragalus and 90
    olive leaf and 156–57
folic acid 57–59
    birth defects and 58
    food sources of 59
Food and Drug Administration 10
free radicals 113, 175–76, 208
Garlic 147–52
    immune function and 148–49
    heart disease and 148–49
    ulcers and 150–51
    antioxidant properties of 151
    as antibiotic 150–51
gastrointestinal health
    probiotics and 85
    fiber and 117–19
genetic material 58–59
genistein (see "isoflavones")
ginkgo 209
glucomannan 120
glutathione 66
glucosamine 208
Glyconutrients 93–105
    immunity and 94–98
    autoimmune disorders and 98–100
    cancer and 100–01
    chronic fatigue and 101
    candidiasis and 104
    fibromyalgia and 104
    lupus and 99
    rheumatoid arthritis and 99–100
    sources of 102–103
grapefruit seed extract 211
Grapeseed extract 175–182
    antioxidant properties of 176–79
    heart disease and 177, 180–81
    multiple sclerosis and 177–79
    anti-inflammatory effect of 179
    vascular system and 180–81
    vision and 181
    aging problems and 180–82
Green foods 197–206
    disease prevention and 197–201
    supplement forms of 204–205
    immune function and 203
    juicing and 204–05

Green tea 125–31
    antioxidant properties of 126–28
    cancer and 128–29
    immunity and 130
    heart disease and 128–31
guggul 209
H. pylori 150–51
hawthorn 211
heart disease 36, 44, 54, 64, 211, 212
    niacin and 64

beta carotene and 116
fiber and 120–21, 123
green tea and 128–31
isoflavones and 144
garlic and 148–49
olive leaf and 158
grapeseed extract and 177
natural progesterone and 187–88
hepatitis B 103
hepatitis C 103
high blood pressure 130–31, 209
Hippocrates 109
hormone replacement therapy (HRT) 140, 183–86
hot flashes 140
homocysteine 57
hyperimmune egg 209
hypoglycemia 158–59
immune function 57, 208, 209, 210
echinacea and 71–75
probiotics and 78–85
glyconutrients and 97–98
beta carotene and 110–11
green tea 130
insomnia 210
Isoflavones 139–46
menopause and 140
cancer and 141–42
PMS and 142–43
heart disease and 144
osteoporosis and 144
Journal of the American Medical Association 183

kidney stones 55
lactose intolerance 85
L-arginine 212
lipoic acid 212
liver health 211
lupus 36, 44, 99
lycopene 208
magnesium 30
manganese 31
menopause 140
natural progesterone and 183–95
mental function 61–63, 209
methylsulfonylmethane (MSM) 210
migraines 44, 66–67
milk thistle 211
minerals 28
trace mineral supplements 28
multiple sclerosis 44
Multivitamin-Mineral supplements 19–33
benefits of 20–21
guaranteed potency of 16
guidelines for 22–32
quality control of 24–25
mushrooms, medicinal 104
niacin 63–64
nutrient, malabsorption of 85
oat bran 121–22
obesity 119
oleuropein 154
oligomeric proanthocyanidins (OPCs) 176–78

Index

Olive leaf 153–60
    anti-microbial activity of 154–57
    cold/flu and 156–157
    heart disease and 158
    diabetes and 158–59
omega-3 fats (see essential fatty acids)
omega-6 fats 46
oral disease 130
osteoporosis 144
    calcium and 168–70
    natural progesterone and 191–92
pantothenic acid 60–61
passionflower 210
pectin 121
PEPI trial 184
pharmaceutical drugs 10
"phyto"-foods (see "green foods")
polysaccharides (see "glyconutrients")
potassium 30
Premarin 185
premenstrual syndrome (PMS) 142–43, 192
Probiotics 77–86
    forms of 80–81
    guidelines for 82–85
Progesterone, natural 183–95
    compared to synthetic hormone treatment 185–86
    heart disease and 187–88
    breast cancer and 188–90
    mental function and 191
    osteoporosis and 191–92
    PMS and 192
    natural estrogen and 193–94
    wild yam as "progesterone" 193
Prometrium 186
prostate health 161–65
Provera 185
psyllium 120–21
Rhodiola rosea 207–08
riboflavin 66–67
St. John's wort 210
Saw palmetto 161–66
    BPH and 163–66
    infertility in women and 163
    comparison to drugs 165–66

Schweitzer, Albert 147
selenium 31
seroctin 211
sexual function 166, 194, 211, 212
skin problems 211
soy 139–146
soy isoflavones (see "isoflavones")
stress 210
supplements
    tips for choosing 14–16
thiamin 61–63
transfer factor 208
ulcers 179–80
valerian 210
vascualr system 180–81
vision 181, 209
Vitamin A (see also "beta

carotene") 27, 107–116
Vitamin B complex 29, 51–67
    summary of 62
vitamin B6 53–55
vitamin B12 55–57
Vitamin C 27, 35–42
    benefits of 36
    free radicals and 38–39
    megadosing 40–41
    energy and 41–42
vitamin D 29
vitamin E 28–29
vitamin K 29
weight management 119–20, 208
wild yam 193
yeast infection, chronic 79, 211
zinc 31